Praise for
Experts' Guide

"We are at a critical point in history where women are taking more and more control over their careers and futures – but fertility is more complicated than ever. As we're having kids later in life, it's essential to get clinical, unbiased information about reproductive health even before we're thinking abouts kids. Dr. Lamb's book does a terrific job of boiling down all the conversations surrounding egg freezing so women have a go-to resource for learning about the procedure, success rates, advantages, and risks. This comprehensive view is key for any woman considering fertility treatments."
– *Afton Vechery, co-founder and CEO of Modern Fertility*

"This book explains clearly what you need to know about freezing your eggs. As a reproductive endocrinologist who counsels women everyday about egg freezing and how to maximize their fertility and reproductive health, I highly recommend this book! It will be a great resource to you as you decide whether egg freezing is right for you."
– *Dr. Serena Chen, Director of Reproductive Medicine and Clinical Associate Professor at IRMS Institute of Reproductive Medicine, Rutgers Robert Wood Johnson Medical School*

"I am thrilled to have this book to give my patients! With a step-by-step review for preparing and actually doing the treatment, this is an excellent guide for anyone considering or preparing for fertility preservation."
– *Lora Shahine, MD, FACOG, author of Not Broken: An Approachable Guide to Miscarriage and Recurrent Pregnancy Loss*

"Dr. Julie Lamb and Emily Gray deliver a must-read book for anyone considering egg freezing for family planning choices. Together the duo lay out step-by-step exactly how egg freezing works, what to plan for and expect from the fertility treatments, and invaluable takeaway tips and tricks for anyone going through a cycle. As a three-time egg freezer myself, this book is what I wish I would have had and known before I started my own egg freezing journey."
– *Valerie Landis, 37-year-old egg freezer, fertility patient advocate, and founder of eggsperience.com*

The Fertility Experts' Guide to Egg Freezing

Everything You Need to Know About Putting Your Fertility on Ice

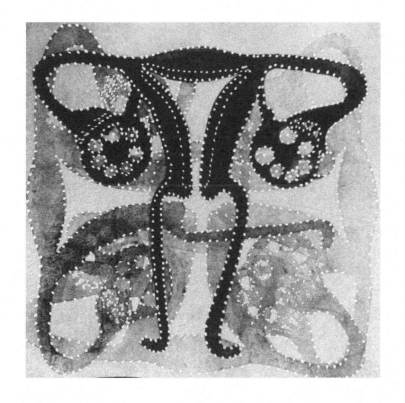

JULIE LAMB, MD
EMILY GRAY, RN, BSN

Seattle, Washington
2020

The Fertility Experts' Guide to Egg Freezing: Everything You Need to Know About Putting Your Fertility on Ice

ISBN: 978-1-7923-4084-0

Dedication

We dedicate this book to all our brave patients. These are the strong women who have lived and breathed the good, the bad, and the ugly of egg freezing. From difficult conversations, uncomfortable work excuses, injections, blood draws, vaginal ultrasounds, needles, mood changes, tears, empowerment, and the unexpected outcomes, egg freezing has it all! We have seen first-hand the strength of our awesome patients, and we applaud them, we cheer them on, and we empower them to take charge of their fertility.

Julie Lamb, MD
Director of Fertility Preservation
Pacific NW Fertility and IVF Specialists
Clinical Faculty, University of Washington

Emily Gray, RN, BSN
Director of IVF Nursing
Pacific NW Fertility and IVF Specialists

Contents

Introduction

So you are considering preserving your fertility. Good for you! Way to take charge of your reproductive potential and plan for your future. Whether you haven't met the right partner, need to focus on school or your career, aren't ready to parent, or have a medical condition that affects fertility, there are many reasons to consider egg freezing. It is liberating and exciting to do so, but it is still a large undertaking, and you need to educate yourself and go in with eyes wide open.

Why is it important to learn about fertility? Get ready for yet another big gender inequity, as if there weren't already enough. Did you know that a woman is born with all the eggs she will ever have and that the number of eggs and the quality of her eggs declines over time, more significantly after age 35? By age 40, 50% of women have difficulty achieving pregnancy, and by age 45, 99% of women are infertile. The number of potential eggs available for pregnancy and the quality of those eggs declines with time until none are remaining at the time of menopause. And while the ovaries age, the uterus doesn't in the same way. So using these eggs earlier in life or saving them by freezing for later use can make a huge difference for women and their ability to achieve their future family goals. Unfortunately, looking and feeling young doesn't equal good fertility, and unintended childlessness is a common consequence of delayed childbearing. So just like you prepare for your financial future by learning, planning, and saving, we are here to encourage you to do the same with your fertility.

Egg freezing provides women with more choices in reproductive health by providing a means to "stop the biological clock," essentially a technological bridge from biological reproductive prime to preferred age of conception. Through the ovarian stimulation portion of IVF (in vitro fertilization), women grow follicles and mature eggs that can be removed from the ovary, frozen, and saved for later use. Many people are choosing to delay pregnancy until later in their 30s and 40s in today's society due to work, finances, and social circumstances. Unfortunately, evolution hasn't caught up to this cultural shift. Fertility potential does decline with age, meaning egg freezing can be a way for women to feel empowered to act now in an attempt to avoid infertility when trying to conceive later in life.

Experience matters when it comes to egg freezing, as the technology that allows for the successful freezing and thawing of eggs is relatively new. It is important to research and find a clinic that has had success and ample experience in the vitrification (freezing) of eggs. Whether you are committed to fertility preservation or you are still deciding if it's right for you, we're here to help. We'll start by reviewing many aspects of fertility preservation, including fertility testing and the ovarian stimulation process, and will help you better understand your own fertility potential. We will also include information about what's next – how to use those eggs in the future (if you need to) and what this process may look like for you.

Egg freezing isn't easy – it takes a lot of time, energy, and money. Stimulation begins with roughly two weeks of injectable medications (yes, with needles), several vaginal ultrasounds, and blood draws to prepare the ovaries for a surgical procedure with light sedation where the eggs are removed (though a needle in your vagina!). There can be plenty of side effects, but the main ones are bloating and fatigue. The two largest drawbacks of egg freezing are the cost (like all medical treatment, it is expensive, and it is often not covered by insurance) and the fact that the eggs might not work in the future (lack of a guarantee). Reproductive biology is very inefficient, and in some cases, you can save a lot of eggs and still not have enough to make a baby when you go to use them. Each patient is unique, and success of treatment varies widely case by case. This can make the success of egg freezing difficult to predict in advance (at the time of freezing), which is challenging for many women as they evaluate if they have saved enough eggs to build their future family.

So now that you know some of the basics, what are the next steps in taking charge of your fertility? This book will help you learn about the egg freezing process and help you better understand what testing is done and how to interpret it for your cycle and overall reproductive potential. It will review side effects, tips/tricks to success, and even the common mistakes many people make. It is not meant to take the place of a conversation with a fertility specialist, or give you any medical advice. It is a field guide to help you navigate the process, but please realize that no two people's bodies are the same and that everyone's experience is somewhat different. Egg freezing can be empowering and a little freeing from the constraints of natural fertility, but it's not always easy. In fact, while most of our patients dread the needles and worry about mood swings, it is often less physically demanding and more emotionally demanding than anticipated. The process of egg freezing can be as emotionally exhausting as the process of infertility may potentially be in the future. Feelings of frustration, anger, sadness, blame, and isolation can occur. Feeling comfortable talking with your support system, your provider and/or nurse, a counselor or other professional, or a peer support group in your area can help. Most importantly, remember – you are not alone!

Disclaimer: This book does not replace the advice of your doctor. It is meant as a resource and a helping hand and should not be taken as medical advice.

– Julie Lamb, MD, and Emily Gray, RN, BSN

1
Fertility 101: How Fertility Changes With Age and What It All Means

The number of births in the United States is at its lowest level in 30 years. The National Center for Health Statistics reports that the US fertility rate fell in every reproductive age group, except in women aged 40-44. This reflects a new generation of women who are delaying childbearing for all sorts of reasons – whether it's to pursue more education, to climb the corporate ladder, because they just aren't ready to parent, or maybe, most commonly, because they just haven't found the partner they want to parent with yet. Regardless, these delays are creating a cultural shift toward family building later in life.

In just one generation, we moved from childbearing in our 20s to having kids in our late 30s or even early 40s. And this change has resulted in more women having significantly more difficulty building their ideal families. Did you know that by age 40, 50% of women have difficulty conceiving? Just one more thing in the long list of gender inequities is that men make new sperm every day, but women are born with all the eggs they will ever have. By 35, half a woman's eggs are abnormal, and by 40, it approaches 80%. This means if a woman is waiting until her late 30s, each egg is less likely to cause a pregnancy – increasing both the time to conception and the risk of miscarriage.

It used to be that a woman would wait until she was having difficulty conceiving to seek out help from a fertility specialist. If she was unable to conceive with her own eggs, she might move to donor eggs – using eggs from a younger woman to achieve pregnancy. While a woman's eggs age, a woman's uterus really doesn't. And while using donor eggs is no one's first choice, this option allows for a healthy pregnancy when the current set of eggs is no longer working. Using donor eggs, however, means that although you have some biological link to the child when you carry the pregnancy, you don't have the direct genetic link that comes from using the DNA of your own egg. In comes egg freezing, which potentially solves this problem by allowing the proactive preservation of eggs with your own genetic material. This process allows women to save some of their own eggs for potential future pregnancies in case their own eggs aren't working when they are ready to conceive down the road.

2
The Hormone Madness: Understanding the Menstrual Cycle

To understand the fertility preservation cycle, an understanding of the natural menstrual cycle is helpful. A menstrual cycle is counted from the first day of a period (full flow bleeding, not including spotting) to the first day of the subsequent period. An average cycle is roughly 28 days long but can range in length for each woman and is considered pretty typical when it ranges from about 24-35 days (from the beginning of one period to the beginning of the next).

A menstrual cycle consists of two phases. First, the follicular phase begins with day one of a menstrual cycle and lasts for roughly the 14 days it takes to grow and mature an egg within a follicle (a fluid-filled sac that is measured by ultrasound and houses the microscopic egg). The predominant hormone in this phase of the cycle is estrogen, which is produced by the developing follicle and causes the lining of the uterus (the endometrium) to grow and thicken to get ready for the possibility of implantation. The day of ovulation varies significantly between individuals but involves the release of the egg from the follicle.

The second half of the cycle is the luteal phase, and this phase goes from the time of ovulation until the next cycle day one or when menstruation begins again. It is named for the corpus luteum, which is the structure that results from the follicle after the egg is released. This half of the cycle is progesterone dominant, and this hormone readies the uterine lining (endometrium) for potential implantation. The egg that was released during ovulation moves down the fallopian tube to meet with sperm if fertilization is to occur. When fertilization occurs, implantation can then happen, and the embryo buries itself in the uterine lining. If fertilization does not occur, menstruation begins and the unfertilized egg will pass with the shedding of the endometrial/uterine lining.

Without implantation, progesterone levels that spiked after ovulation eventually drop and result in the shedding of the uterine lining when your period begins. If implantation happens, then the hCG (human chorionic gonadotropin) hormone produced by the pregnancy stimulates the corpus luteum (what the follicle turns into after the egg is released) to continue progesterone and estrogen production. Continued production maintains the uterine lining and thus supports the developing pregnancy until the placenta takes over this hormonal production between six to eight weeks of pregnancy.

Some hormonal variations can result in a disruption of the menstrual cycle. These include ovulation dysfunction, PCOS (polycystic ovarian syndrome), abnormalities in prolactin or thyroid levels, and more. Make sure to seek medical attention if you have irregular cycles or questions about your menstrual cycle.

3
What to Expect at Your Appointment

The First Step: The Initial Appointment

By making an appointment and considering fertility preservation, you have made the first big step. Just by contacting a clinic and provider, you are learning more about your options, educating yourself, and being an advocate for your own future fertility. You have choices in where you receive your care, so choose a clinic that will help you achieve your goals. Experience has never mattered more – make sure to choose a leader in egg freezing and IVF.

What to Expect: Getting Started

Prior to your first visit, you will be asked to register as a patient with the clinic, and records on any prior testing or gynecologic history will be requested. At your first appointment, your health history will be reviewed – including any medical history, surgical history, allergies, and medications you may be taking. You will also be asked about any prior pregnancies, the regularity or irregularity of your cycles, types of birth control used, and whether you have pain with your period or any history of pelvic infections. Your provider may also ask you about family history of endometriosis or early menopause. It's important to give an accurate history, so if there is something unusual about a prior surgery or something that happened in childhood, make sure to ask your family or request records before you go so you can get the story straight.

This is also your chance to tell the doctor about yourself and what your goals and fears are and to really make sure they understand who you are. For example, if you are starting a seven-year PhD program, want four kids someday, or your mom went through menopause at 38, these are all the kinds of things that a provider would want to know as they could potentially affect your personal fertility plan. Also, if you have done previous fertility testing or treatment, make sure to let them know.

Some patients have specific medical reasons to consider egg freezing, and those should be discussed at this initial appointment. These could include a history of ovarian surgery, recurrent ovarian cysts, a history of endometriosis or pelvic infections, a genetic predisposition to early menopause, a plan to initiate treatment for gender dysphoria, or cancer requiring treatment that could compromise fertility. Make sure to let your doctor know if there is something that you believe could compromise your future fertility.

Next, you will discuss fertility testing. This often includes a vaginal ultrasound and blood work. The timing of the fertility testing is dependent on your menstrual cycle – so it may take up to a month (or more) for you to get these tests completed. (Please refer to Chapters 4 and 5 for more information on pre-cycle testing and how to interpret results). At this initial appointment, you will also learn a little about what you can expect during the process of egg freezing (see Chapters 7 and 8 for all the details).

Once your fertility testing is complete, you will have a little better idea of what you might expect from your egg freezing cycle. Remember, these test results don't define you. Unfortunately, you can't work or study harder to make them better. These tests can be better than, as good as, or not as good as your doctor was hoping to see. The results are used to help your doctor counsel you about how efficient egg freezing might be for you, as well as how many eggs you might be able to expect from the stimulation process. These tests also help to make a recommendation for a personalized treatment plan, including a medication protocol and dosing.

Timeline Overview

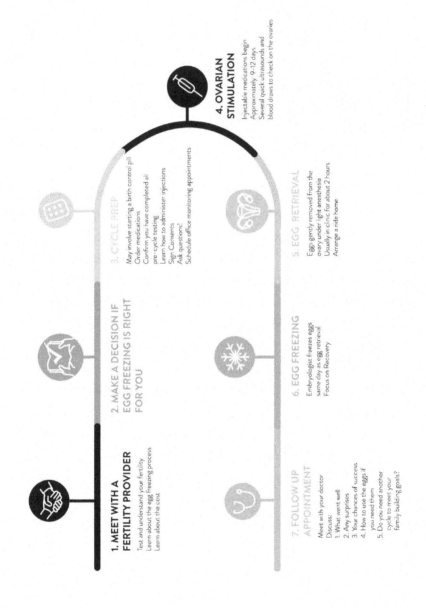

1. MEET WITH A FERTILITY PROVIDER

Test and understand your fertility
Learn about the egg freezing process
Learn about the cost

2. MAKE A DECISION IF EGG FREEZING IS RIGHT FOR YOU

3. CYCLE PREP

May involve starting a birth control pill
Order medications
Confirm you have completed all pre-cycle testing
Learn how to administer injections
Sign Consents
Ask questions!
Schedule office monitoring appointments

4. OVARIAN STIMULATION

Injectable medications begin
Approximately 9-12 days
Several quick ultrasounds and blood draws to check on the ovaries

5. EGG RETRIEVAL

Eggs gently removed from the ovary under light anesthesia
Usually in clinic for about 2 hours
Arrange a ride home

6. EGG FREEZING

Embryologist freezes eggs same day as egg retrieval
Focus on Recovery

7. FOLLOW UP APPOINTMENT

Meet with your doctor
Discuss:
1. What went well
2. Any surprises
3. Your chances of success
4. How to use the eggs if you need them
5. Do you need another cycle to meet your family building goals?

4
Fertility Testing: Understanding Your Ovarian Reserve

Ovarian reserve testing is a little window into your reproductive potential – imagine it like peeking in on your eggs. Testing typically consists of blood work and a transvaginal ultrasound that helps to better understand your fertility potential, or how efficient the egg freezing process might be for you.

Testing does not tell your provider if you are fertile, or whether or not you could have a baby if you were trying to get pregnant. It does not tell you how likely your eggs are to work if you need them or how many eggs it will take to make a baby. It is the best marker we have prior to stimulating the ovaries to evaluate how many eggs might be available in a given month and how many eggs may be retrieved during a stimulation cycle, but these tests aren't perfect.

Getting a number that is "good for your age" does not guarantee an easy time conceiving or predict how many years you have left to successfully procreate. Similarly, 'bad results' or 'low results' do not mean someone could not conceive if they were actively trying. However, a high FSH (follicle-stimulating hormone) and low AMH (anti-Müllerian hormone) may indicate that the response to fertility treatment (such as egg freezing or IVF) and fertility medications may be lower, and less efficient. Your provider may recommend proceeding with a more aggressive treatment protocol and may recommend undergoing the process sooner rather than waiting longer as values tend to diminish with time.

It is important to understand that age is the largest contributor to egg quality. Fertility declines significantly with age, not just because the quantity of the ovarian reserve supply diminishes, but because the quality of the remaining eggs declines as well. At age 35, half a woman's eggs are genetically normal, but by age 40, the number of abnormal eggs approaches 80%. So with advancing age, it takes more eggs to find the good one (unfortunately, with advancing age, fewer eggs are available as well). For instance, a 44-year-old woman may have reassuring or 'normal' fertility results (quantity), but she still only has a 40% chance of pregnancy when saving eggs or when trying naturally to conceive due to the quality of those remaining eggs, whereas a 34-year-old woman with low egg count test results (low ovarian reserve quantity) has a significantly better chance of pregnancy from frozen eggs, even if she is only able to save a few. This is because a smaller number of eggs is needed to find a good (genetically normal) one for conception at this younger age.

There are three different tests that together give your provider a picture about your ovarian reserve supply and a clue to how you might respond to the stimulation medications.

1. AFC (Antral Follicle Count):

❑ A subjective count of resting follicles on each ovary done with pelvic ultrasound. It is subjective because there's a person looking and counting, and some ovaries are easier to see than others.

❑ In general, a 'normal' antral follicle count is 10-12 follicles total between both ovaries, but these values can vary widely.

❑ Each follicle should contain an egg, and the more follicles, the more eggs available to recruit/develop with fertility treatments and ovarian stimulation.

❑ A high antral follicle count, defined as more than 12 resting (antral) follicles per ovary, can be associated with PCOS (polycystic ovary syndrome). However, a high count alone cannot diagnose PCOS – some women (especially young women) may just have a more robust egg supply. To diagnose PCOS, other factors must also be present.

2. FSH (Follicle-Stimulating Hormone):

❏ This is a hormone secreted from the pituitary gland that encourages the ovaries to recruit an egg to mature and develop in the first half of the menstrual cycle (the follicular phase).

❏ FSH levels are highest in the beginning of the cycle (cycle days two, three, or four) when the estradiol (estrogen) levels in the body are low. The ideal FSH value is <10 mIU/mL when checked in the beginning of a menstrual cycle.

❏ As providers, we check estradiol levels in the blood at the same time as FSH because a high estradiol level will feedback to falsely lower the FSH level – meaning an estradiol level over 80 pg/mL can give a falsely reassuring FSH level of lower than 10. If this happens, it is often recommended to recheck both estradiol (E2) and FSH in a subsequent cycle for an accurate measurement. The estradiol measurement at the time of FSH allows for accuracy and more dependable FSH results.

❏ Estrogen (estradiol or E2) blood levels should be low early in the menstrual cycle. High estradiol levels early in the cycle can be attributed to:

1. A cyst (which is just a leftover follicle) from the previous menstrual cycle that will resolve usually on its own with time.

2. Checking at a different time in the cycle (the patient had bleeding, but it wasn't really the beginning of a menstrual cycle) – meaning the value was done at an inaccurate time in the cycle.

3. Early follicular recruitment (recruiting a follicle too early in the menstrual cycle), which can be an indication of low ovarian reserve. This is more common in women who have short menstrual cycles (<24 days).

❏ FSH can vary from cycle to cycle, and if someone is checking it multiple cycles in a row, then sometimes it can be high and sometimes normal. Studies show that a woman's success with fertility treatment is best predicted by her highest ('worst') FSH. This means that if someone checks FSH three months in a row and one value is 15 mIU/mL and the others <10 (all with estradiol <80), then she is still considered to have diminished or low ovarian reserve.

❏ We cannot fix a high FSH or 'make it better' – it's reflective of ovarian reserve/what's going on in the ovaries. When the FSH value exceeds 10, it means the brain (pituitary) is working harder to develop a follicle each month, or that the ovary may be getting a little bit resistant to the FSH hormone and thus needs higher circulating FSH levels to respond.

❏ We do not recommend repeatedly checking FSH to see if it 'gets better' – rechecking FSH should be used to evaluate if it's getting worse (since the highest FSH predicts success with treatment), and more reassuring values in one cycle do not negate previous results.

FSH	Estradiol	Interpretation
<10 mIU/mL	<80 pg/mL	Reassuring results
10-20 mIU/mL	<80 pg/mL	Diminished ovarian reserve (low egg supply)
>20 mIU/mL	<80 pg/mL	Significant diminished ovarian reserve; less likely to respond favorably to ovarian stimulation

What do we know when FSH is high?

❏ It signals diminished ovarian reserve and may mean fewer good quality eggs remain.

❏ It is found more commonly when someone is having difficulty conceiving.

- ❏ It may explain recurrent miscarriage that is otherwise unexplained (due to conceiving with poor quality eggs).
- ❏ It can mean a lower success rate with any fertility treatment.
- ❏ It may mean that the fertility window is shorter (it doesn't tell us how long someone has until menopause).
- ❏ It may mean you want to be more aggressive when trying to save eggs for the future.
- ❏ It may mean that your chances of success with saving eggs for the future is low enough that you will want to make other plans for building your family (for instance, a donor egg).

3. AMH (Anti-Müllerian Hormone):

- ❏ A hormone produced by supporting cells around the eggs in the ovaries that will be available that month.
- ❏ In general, the higher the AMH, the higher the number of eggs there are in reserve, and the more that can be retrieved in a single cycle.
- ❏ AMH is a quantitative measure of ovarian reserve and can be considered a more objective (and more easily measured) form of the antral follicle count (counting follicles with transvaginal ultrasound).
- ❏ AMH is a window into future fertility. When low, there is concern that the window of fertility could be shorter than what is predicted by age alone.
- ❏ AMH declines with age, and in general:

Age	Expected/Average
20s	3.0-4.0 ng/mL
30-34	2.0-3.0 ng/mL
35-39	1.0-2.0 ng/mL
40	1.0 ng/mL

41+	<1.0 ng/mL

A high AMH:

❏ An AMH >5 can be associated with PCOS, but it is not diagnostic – some women just have a higher ovarian reserve.

❏ Super high AMHs >10 are not extremely accurate – the blood work assay (measurement in the lab) gets less reliable with high levels, and anything over eight is considered to be just 'very high ovarian reserve.'

❏ A higher AMH can predict a higher recruitment of eggs with fertility treatment and guides us to use a lower dose or different medications for the ovarian stimulation.

❏ A high AMH can indicate a higher risk of OHSS (ovarian hyperstimulation syndrome) with a fertility preservation cycle and helps us choose protocols to decrease that risk and keep patients safe (please see Chapter 15 for more information about OHSS).

A low AMH (defined as an AMH <1.0):

❏ A low AMH is often called diminished ovarian reserve (DOR), no matter what your age.

❏ A low AMH often means a higher dose of gonadotropins may be recommended for your protocol in order to stimulate as many eggs as possible during a cycle.

❏ A low AMH does not predict someone's ability to conceive naturally.

❏ A low AMH does not predict when you will run out of eggs or your age of menopause (charts online where you plug in a current age and AMH value and get a predicted age of menopause are not reliable!).

❏ A low AMH often means a lower number of eggs retrieved with ovarian stimulation, which can mean a lower chance of success with eggs in the future, because there are fewer of them to start.

❏ A low AMH may mean you will likely need to plan for more than one egg freezing cycle in order to achieve your goal number of frozen eggs.

❏ A low AMH may predict a lower response to the egg freezing medications and an increased chance of deciding to cancel the cycle due to no response or a suboptimal response to the stimulation medications.

Breaking It Down: Egg Supply Equations

❏ *Ovarian reserve* = egg supply = a combination of FSH, AMH (blood tests), and AFC (by transvaginal ultrasound)

❏ *"Good" egg supply* = ⇓FSH (<10 mIU/mL), ⇑AMH (>1-2 ng/mL), and ⇑AFC (>10-12)

❏ *"Less good" egg supply* = ⇑FSH (>10 mIU/mL), ⇓AMH (<1 ng/mL), and ⇓AFC (<10-12)

5

My Head Is Spinning – What Does This All Mean? Interpreting Ovarian Reserve

Interpreting ovarian reserve testing really depends on *why* you are testing:

Why are you testing?	Reassuring results FSH <10 mIU/mL AMH >1-2 ng/mL	Diminished ovarian reserve (DOR) FSH >10 mIU/mL and/or AMH <1.0 ng/mL
Trying to conceive	Does not mean every egg is perfect, but reassuring that there are good eggs left!	Can explain one reason why it is taking a long time to conceive. Fewer good quality eggs available.
Planning fertility treatment	Success rates are most likely consistent with general success rates with age.	Success rates with any fertility treatment will be lower than expected for age as there are fewer good eggs in reserve.
Planning egg freezing/ fertility preservation	Reassuring – counseling for outcomes and predicting the number of eggs to preserve will depend on age and AMH level.	Patients may need to plan for more than one egg freezing cycle to retrieve a reassuring number of eggs.

What if my results are really 'abnormal for my age'?

If the FSH is >15 and/or the AMH is <0.5:

- ❏ Know that nothing is ever based on only one level – it is always okay to recheck.
- ❏ Remember that abnormal ovarian reserve numbers do not mean someone cannot conceive if they are currently trying.
- ❏ Be careful of what you read on the internet – it's always okay to educate yourself, but remember that not everything you find online is true.
- ❏ Write down questions to review with your doctor.
- ❏ Sometimes women's priorities change from fertility preservation to an active attempt to conceive sooner when ovarian reserve is lower than anticipated.
- ❏ Lower ovarian reserve numbers help set expectations that egg freezing may be less efficient. These numbers help us warn you about higher cancellation rates for asynchronous follicular growth or no growth at all and likelihood of fewer eggs at the time of an egg retrieval. No test is the perfect predictor, and you could easily get more than you anticipate. You may decide to do more than one cycle. You should anticipate fewer eggs than your same-aged peers who have more 'normal' levels.
- ❏ Everyone benefits from learning about the option of donor eggs. This is when you use an egg from a younger woman to conceive when you are ready. While it is not typically a first choice, it provides another option for family building that can be much more efficient when one's own egg supply is very low. Some women decide to bypass the struggle of ovarian stimulation for fertility preservation and will plan to use a donated egg if unable to conceive when ready.

Key points about ovarian reserve testing:

1. These numbers do NOT tell you if you are fertile or infertile.

2. Getting ovarian reserve testing can be emotional – it touches on all sorts of issues that are important related to the idea of building your future family. Don't let it define you.
3. Knowledge is power. It's important to know these numbers so you can make informed choices about your health.
4. It's important to stay realistic.
5. How women make choices about these numbers varies widely, and that is okay. Some women will decide not to save eggs for the future if it's only a 50% chance, while other women want to try even if it's a <5% chance. The important part is that it's your choice. No doctor or friend can decide what's right for you.

6
Preparing Your Body for Egg Freezing: Vitamins, Exercise, Stress, and Eliminating Toxins

There are a lot of unknowns about how environmental toxins, stress, and nutrition potentially influence fertility. Therefore, the general recommendation is to be your healthiest self when preparing for egg freezing so that whatever the outcome, you know you did everything possible to optimize your success.

Target a Healthy Body Weight

Having a body mass index (BMI) that is higher or lower than normal can affect many aspects of your overall health, including your reproductive health. BMI is calculated by dividing your weight in kilograms by your height squared in meters (you can easily find a calculator online). Being overweight (BMI 25-30), obese (BMI >30), or underweight (BMI <19) can affect fertility, and is associated with an increased risk for difficulty conceiving. There are also procedural and anesthesia risks that increase with increasing BMI. Being a healthy weight improves your response to IVF medications and may improve egg freezing outcomes. When overweight or obese, even a small improvement in BMI can improve fertility outcomes. Talk to your doctor about what goals might be right for you.

Minimize Stress

Stress can make the process of egg freezing more anxiety-provoking and can amplify the side effects you may experience. Make sure to minimize work and other social stressors as much as possible. Introduce stress reduction practices such as exercise, journaling, mindfulness, meditation, and calming yoga. Don't underestimate the power of positive thinking! Try to adopt a positive mindset and surround yourself with positive people. Build a support system that includes someone who knows you and you feel comfortable sharing the egg freezing process with. This could be a parent, a partner, a friend, a fellow egg freezer, or a co-worker. Choose someone who could potentially drive you home after the procedure, someone who you find to be encouraging and uplifting.

It isn't possible to eliminate all life stressors, but if you are feeling particularly stressed or anxious about the process, consider establishing care with a mental health professional. This has been shown to support women though the egg freezing or IVF process.

Remember, we are used to working hard and getting the results that we want. To have something so outside of our control, where a certain result is not guaranteed, can be a source of stress for many. Try not to stress about stress – do your best to minimize extra triggers, but know that life is never completely stress free – do your best!

Exercise

Regular, moderate exercise improves overall health. Thirty minutes per day at least four days a week should be part of your routine to prepare your body for your egg freezing cycle. Exercise is a wonderful way to keep your body healthy, your blood flowing, and your mind clear.

In general, during your egg freezing cycle, you want to avoid all high impact exercises, including contact sports, heavy lifting, and high intensity workouts. These recommendations are due to the discomfort related to significant and rapid growth of the ovaries, fluid shifts in the body that can occur with this growth, and the small chance that an ovary could turn on its blood supply (torsion), which is a very rare but significant complication. Low impact activities such as walking, elliptical training, and yoga (without inversions) are okay to continue throughout the stimulation cycle. It is not uncommon to feel your ovaries in your lower abdomen as they start to grow, especially when being active. Listen to your body – if exercise becomes uncomfortable, be sure to adjust your activities or stop. In fact, you may not feel like exercising at all, but continuing low-impact activities that are not uncomfortable can improve your sleep, mood, and recovery.

Do not hesitate to talk to your doctor about how to appropriately modify your specific exercise routine around the time of your egg retrieval.

Nutrition

As you prepare for your egg freezing cycle, make sure to eat a healthy diet. You can start by minimizing processed foods. Try to increase foods that are in their natural state and avoid foods with labels that include a long list of ingredients (as these are likely processed). Increase whole foods, specifically organic fruits and veggies. Fruits and vegetables should make up at least half of your plate with each meal. There is no one diet that is proven to improve fertility or your egg quality, but a nutritious and well-balanced diet may be helpful.

Minimize or Eliminate Alcohol

Alcohol is known to negatively influence male and female reproductive systems and the unborn fetus, yet its influence on fertility is not yet well understood. Current recommendations are to completely eliminate alcohol when pregnant or when trying to conceive. We encourage our patients to minimize alcohol for one to three months prior to their egg freezing cycle and eliminate alcohol during their stimulation cycle.

Vitamins/Supplements

You should be able to get all your nutrients from a healthy diet, but patients often ask about additional supplementation. Here is a short list (in alphabetic order) of supplements you could consider adding to your healthy diet that some data implies may improve fertility outcomes, but make sure to check in with your doctor first about which of these supplements might be right for you.

❏ **DHEA**: A steroid hormone that may improve the quantity of eggs in women with decreased egg supply. Note: DHEA can be associated with side effects such as acne and hair growth.

❏ **Folic acid**: Included in prenatal vitamins, folic acid may be important for egg quality and fertility in addition to pregnancy health.

❏ **Melatonin**: An antioxidant and anti-inflammatory that helps regulate the sleep/wake cycles (circadian rhythm).

❏ **Myo-inositol**: A vitamin B component of the cell membrane that may improve IVF outcomes for patients with PCOS.

❏ **Omega-3 fatty acids (DHA)**: DHA may improve the health of the reproductive system by decreasing inflammation.

❏ **Ubiquinol**: A more absorbable form of CoQ10, ubiquinol is an antioxidant that may improve egg quality and chromosomal division.

❏ **Vitamin C**: An antioxidant that helps reduce free radicals.

❏ **Vitamin D**: A fat-soluble vitamin that may improve IVF outcomes.

❏ **Vitamin E**: A fat-soluble antioxidant that may prevent cell membrane damage from free radicals.

If you are taking any herbal supplements or fertility-focused vitamins, we recommend reviewing with your doctor prior to starting the stimulation medications due to any potential and not well understood interactions with the egg freezing medications.

Reduce Environmental Toxins

Some things you can do to minimize toxins prior to your egg freezing cycle:

1. **Don't smoke** or be around people who smoke.
2. **Choose organic** when possible in order to minimize exposure to pesticides.
3. **Take off your shoes** or wipe them well on a doormat to avoid bringing pesticides and other chemicals into your home.

4. **Limit fragrances** and other chemicals in personal hygiene products and make-up.
5. **Limit plastics**, especially in food storage, as this will help decrease exposure to BPA.
6. **Evaluate cleaning products** and make choices that have fewer toxins.
7. **Reduce mercury** exposure by decreasing or eliminating potentially contaminated fish.
8. **Minimize your exposure to VOCs** by using non-toxic building materials and paints.

A toxin-free life is impossible, but making small, meaningful changes to your everyday life to limit toxins may be helpful in improving egg quality and overall health. There is no one thing that makes your follicles grow or not grow, or your eggs work one day or not work another. Continue to educate yourself on the biggest offenders, and aim to take steps to lessen your exposure. It is important to know that you did everything within your control to achieve the best outcome for you.

7

The Ovarian Stimulation Cycle

IVF stands for in vitro fertilization, but in egg freezing, you don't fertilize the eggs now, you freeze them for later. However, the process of growing follicles and maturing the eggs inside you is the same, and that part is called the 'ovarian stimulation' cycle. In other words, that same type of ovarian stimulation cycle can be used for fertility preservation or for IVF when conception is the goal.

The process of egg freezing involves ovarian stimulation using injectable hormonal medications to promote the growth of more follicles (fluid-filled sacs in the ovary that likely contain an egg) to mature during one cycle than would normally occur during a natural cycle. Since not every egg results in a baby, this allows us to try to get more eggs from a single cycle. Every month, you naturally ovulate one egg, and a small group of eggs dies away. Ovarian stimulation organizes the follicles and tries to get that entire group of potentially available eggs to mature together inside of you to take advantage of more eggs that would otherwise be lost that cycle.

An egg freezing cycle can start with birth control pills for a relatively short amount of time leading up to the injection phase. The intention of the pill is not only to prevent pregnancy, but to briefly suppress the ovaries in order to organize the small antral follicles and prevent a dominant one from coming forward – thus producing a cohort of follicles with similar sizes. This can help the follicles grow together at a similar rate once injectable medications have started. While birth control pills seem counterproductive, they can actually help get more mature eggs during an egg freezing cycle. The birth control pill can also be helpful for planning the start of the stimulation cycle.

There are also circumstances where the cycle is started without the use of birth control pills. If a doctor has told you not to take the birth control pill for a health reason, make sure to let your provider know. There are many ways to manipulate the menstrual cycle to give you the best chance of success with your egg freezing cycle, and your doctor will help you decide what the best protocol is for you.

Preparation Phase

During the preparation phase, pre-cycle testing will need to be completed, consents will be signed, ultrasound visits will be scheduled, and egg freezing medications will be ordered through a specialty fertility pharmacy. Egg freezing medications are absorbed through the bloodstream and are administered as injections, often multiple times a day. They mimic your body's natural hormones – just in much larger quantities than in a natural menstrual cycle – in order to recruit and grow more follicles during ovarian stimulation.

Baseline Ultrasound

At the end of the preparation phase, a baseline ultrasound is performed in addition to an estrogen blood test to confirm that the ovaries are ready to start. This is also sometimes called the suppression check, and it is the 'ready, set, go' appointment of your stimulation cycle. If everything looks perfect to start (meaning your ovaries are quiet with no large follicle and the estrogen level is low), stimulation injections will then begin. If your ovary has a dominant hormone-producing follicle or cyst, this may make the other follicles less sensitive to the expensive medications and ultimately impact the success of the cycle. If for some reason it doesn't look perfect to begin with, your doctor may delay the start of stimulation medications until the ovaries are quiet. Starting the injections at the optimal point in the menstrual cycle (usually when all other hormone levels are low and suppressed and antral follicles are small) promotes the highest chance of success in the cycle and the largest quantity of eggs to safely develop.

Maturing the Eggs

The stimulation phase (maturing the eggs) is approximately a two-week process, with daily injections (typically two to three injections a day) and two to five in-office appointments, depending on the ovaries' rate of growth. The appointments typically include a transvaginal ultrasound and often a blood draw. The timing of these visits can fluctuate and are often difficult to predict, particularly toward the end of the stimulation cycle. Plan to be in town and limit commitments both at work and in your personal life during this time. This helps make it less stressful to organize your life around the appointments and allows more time for rest in case you are not feeling well. Most people do very well, with minimal side effects, but the most common symptoms during this stage of the process are bloating and fatigue. It is nice to plan extra rest into your schedule.

This is also the time to really minimize and eventually eliminate intense exercise. The exact recommendations regarding exercise vary based on your stimulation, how you are feeling, the size of your ovaries, and your typical activity level. This is not the time to start a new exercise regimen, but you also don't need to be a couch potato. Listen to your body – if it says to rest, then rest. If you need to move, then consider taking a walk instead of going for a run. Make sure to discuss your specific exercise plan with your medical team.

The intention of the ultrasounds during the stimulation phase of your egg freezing cycle is to monitor the size and rate of growth of the developing follicles. Your doctor is watching to make sure the cohort is growing together and deciding when to start the "antagonist" medication (if that is part of your protocol). (See Chapter 13 for more details on egg freezing medications).

Toward the end of the cycle, the ultrasounds and blood work are to determine the optimal time to administer the "trigger shot" medication, which will determine the day and time of your egg retrieval procedure. The timing of the trigger shot is typically based on follicular size and estradiol blood levels and is important in maximizing the overall success of your egg freezing cycle.

The Egg Retrieval

Once your follicles are "ready" and have reached the right size by ultrasound, your egg retrieval procedure will be scheduled. Typically, your provider can predict a three- to four-day window of when your retrieval will most likely be. As you get closer to your procedure, your provider can give you a little better approximation of when the retrieval will fall. The actual day of your retrieval depends on your ovaries and will be officially determined just two days prior to your procedure – when it's time for the "trigger" shot.

When your follicles are ready, you will be directed to perform a very specifically timed injection to complete the final maturation of the eggs. This "trigger" shot will be timed perfectly with your egg retrieval procedure, which is scheduled typically 35 or 36 hours after administration of the trigger shot. The egg retrieval procedure is performed by a reproductive endocrinologist physician and is often done under anesthesia. Because the timing is determined by follicular growth and because there are many biological differences, the exact date of the procedure is very individualized. So the length of time on injections can vary from person to person and even from cycle to cycle. No one cycle is the same. Usually, your last injection is the evening of your trigger shot (35-36 hours prior to your procedure).

Eggs are collected (retrieved) by ultrasound-guided needle aspiration. A needle is used to gently drain the fluid out of each follicle. With the fluid comes the egg(s). The embryologist will then look through the follicular fluid under the microscope in a temperature-controlled incubator to find each egg. Eggs are studied under the microscope, and the mature eggs are cryopreserved (frozen) for future use. The eggs are kept frozen in a cryostorage tank at -196°C. The eggs can remain in storage for many years. Depending on the number of eggs frozen and your goals, another cycle may be recommended. (For more information about the egg retrieval procedure, refer to Chapter 8).

8
What You Need to Know for Your Big Day: The Egg Retrieval Procedure

The egg (oocyte) retrieval is a procedure in which eggs are removed from the ovaries at the conclusion of an egg freezing cycle. Often, you undergo light anesthesia during the procedure – not heavy, just enough that you will not experience pain during the procedure. A transvaginal ultrasound probe is used to visualize the ovaries, and a needle is passed through the top of the vagina into the ovaries under ultrasound guidance. Gentle suction is applied to collect the follicular fluid and retrieve the eggs. The eggs and fluid from the follicles are collected in heated test tubes and passed to a waiting embryologist, who looks under the microscope to find your eggs. No one likes a needle in their vagina, which is why this procedure is often done under anesthesia. After the procedure, you will know how many eggs were collected from your ovaries. Often by the next day, you will know how many eggs were mature and frozen for you. Only mature eggs are capable of being fertilized, thus the immature eggs are not typically frozen.

The procedure is timed precisely, so it is very important to be on time, even early for your procedure. Plan to leave lots of extra time to minimize stress. Typically, you will be at your fertility center for roughly two hours, although the procedure itself is very quick. Arrange to have a responsible adult driver and companion who can transport you to and from your clinic and stay with you for the rest of the day. You cannot take a cab or other rideshare company home by yourself. Plan ahead, and have someone in mind. If you do not have a companion, let your clinic know, as there are companies that can provide this service. Do not plan on going to work or school on the day of the procedure, and arrange time to rest after the procedure.

If anesthesia is being used, do not eat or drink anything after midnight the night before your procedure. This includes food and liquids, even water. If you take daily oral medications, review with your clinic the recommendations of use on the day of the egg retrieval procedure. On the day of your procedure, be sure to wear comfortable clothing and glasses instead of contacts (if applicable), leave your jewelry at home, and wear warm socks (the procedure rooms can be cold!).

You will be monitored after the procedure to ensure you can urinate and have good pain control before you are able to go home to rest. For the remainder of the day, do not drive, do not go to work or school, do not be the sole caretaker of a child, do not drink alcohol, and have someone stay with you if possible. Make sure to rest more than you normally would, and do something you enjoy.

Most patients recover very quickly from the egg retrieval procedure, but remember that everyone is different. Often women are surprised by how well they feel. If you do have more severe symptoms, remember, they are temporary, and they should continue to improve each day. Stay in contact with your team for encouragement and what to expect if you aren't feeling well. They can often give you tips and tricks to address each symptom. Make sure to stay well hydrated before and after the procedure, as drinking electrolytes can help you feel less tired and bloated. Also, most women will experience a heavier-than-usual period that begins about 7-10 days from the egg retrieval procedure – this can be alarming if you aren't expecting it, but it usually means that you should be feeling better by this point. (For more information on recovery and the days to weeks following the egg retrieval, please refer to Chapter 9).

9

The Egg Freezing Recovery

So you survived the egg retrieval and froze your eggs – that's awesome! What comes next and what happens from the time you leave the egg retrieval until you get a period?

When you get home after your procedure, put on some comfortable clothes, eat a small meal, and park yourself on the couch to rest for the remainder of the day. Remember not to drive, go to work, stay home alone, drink alcohol, or be the sole caretaker of a child. Cramps, abdominal tenderness, and heavy vaginal spotting are common after the procedure and should improve each day.

While most patients return to work the day after their egg retrieval, it often takes 7-10 days for the bloating to resolve completely. Just like in every medical procedure, everyone recovers a little differently. Most doctors recommend ibuprofen (600mg every six hours) to help with possible cramping and discomfort. If you are able to take this for pain, then often you won't require anything stronger. Your doctor may provide you with a prescription for stronger pain medications if needed. Tylenol and other over-the-counter pain medications are also sometimes used after the procedure. Be wary of constipation with pain medications as this can be a common side effect. Over-the-counter stool softeners can be used if needed, and increasing your fluid and fiber intake can also help. To help prevent constipation, some physicians recommend taking a stool softener (Colace 200mg, twice a day) or MiraLAX (over-the-counter), if needed.

After an egg retrieval, it is often recommended to avoid intercourse, tampons, soaking in a bath or hot tub, and high impact exercise for one week following the procedure. Bleeding and spotting can be common after the transvaginal aspiration (TVA) egg retrieval procedure, but if you are soaking more than a pad an hour, let your provider know.

Be sure to contact your clinic if you develop a temperature over 101°F or if you have significant pain, heavy or bright red bleeding, or other concerns. Often, the more eggs you get, the more bloating you will experience. There are huge differences in how people feel and how quickly they recover. Remember to continue to be vigilant about hydration. Protein shakes and electrolyte-enhanced liquids can be helpful, both before and after the procedure. Listen to your body – if you are feeling terrible, then rest more and take care of yourself. Feel free to skip the big work off site, and don't feel like you need to meet up with friends for happy hour or host a dinner party. An egg retrieval is a medical procedure, and it's okay to take a little time off to recover.

Refrain from intense or high impact exercise (like running and contact sports) until all bloating has resolved – this usually takes about a week after the procedure. Avoid using tampons (or putting anything in the vagina) for a week after an egg retrieval procedure. This includes delaying sexual activity for a week as well.

While you are recovering from the egg retrieval procedure, increased rest and self-care are important. Your body is in full recovery mode, the ovaries are still enlarged, and hormone levels are still high until your period begins. Sometimes the symptoms experienced during the ovarian stimulation process can continue after the procedure and can be even more noticeable than during the stimulation phase. Headaches, bloating, fatigue, and cramping are not uncommon. You don't know exactly how you will feel after your egg retrieval, so don't overbook yourself, and schedule in extra time for rest and adequate sleep! Although resting is important, bed rest is not recommended. Walking is a wonderful way to remain active and keep your blood flowing.

Continue to eat as healthy as possible following your procedure. Alcohol, caffeine, and junk food can worsen bloating. Make sure to stay hydrated after your procedure. Some women find that increased electrolyte and protein intake that continues after the egg retrieval can ease recovery by pulling fluid out of the belly and back into circulation. This helps some women feel better quicker (see

Chapter 15 for more information on ovarian hyperstimulation syndrome, or OHSS, and see the recovery summary below for more tips/tricks that may improve bloating).

Constipation is common after the egg retrieval and should be prevented. High levels of progesterone, big fluid shifts in the body, and pain medications can all contribute to worsening constipation post-procedure. Continued hydration, foods high in fiber, stool softeners such as docusate sodium, and MiraLAX (if needed) can all help relieve constipation after the egg retrieval procedure.

Be sure to reach out to your provider's office if you have a fever, worsening pain that is not relieved with medication, heavy bleeding where you are soaking more than a pad an hour, shortness of breath, or other issues that you find concerning. It is much better to reach out than to be home worrying about something, and chances are your care team is familiar with your issue and can offer advice that might help. The majority of women recover easily and quickly following the egg retrieval procedure, but everyone's experience can be very different. Be sure to contact your care team with concerns along the way.

Most women will start a period about 7-10 days after the egg retrieval date. Because your estrogen blood level is higher during a stimulated cycle than in your natural cycle, and you grew more follicles/produced more eggs than a typical menstrual cycle, anticipate this period to be heavier and more crampy than your normal period. This heavier bleeding could include increased flow, passing clots, and/or more days of flow – this is often because of the thick uterine lining that developed due to the high estrogen blood levels while your ovaries were being stimulated. Now that the procedure is behind you, it is okay to use ibuprofen or other over-the-counter pain medications for menstrual cramps as needed!

Recovery Summary

Be sure to speak with your nurse coordinator and provider along your journey and to communicate how you may be feeling.

Getting tips and advice from your care team early on can make a huge difference!

- ❏ Expect bloating and cramping.
- ❏ Anticipate a heavier than usual period in 7-10 days.
- ❏ Do not put anything in your vagina for one week after your egg retrieval procedure.
- ❏ Build extra time into your busy schedule for rest.
- ❏ Avoid caffeine and alcohol as these dehydrate you more.
- ❏ Avoid intense exercise or intercourse while your ovaries are enlarged. Walking is okay, but avoid other intense or high impact exercise.
- ❏ Anticipate constipation – take over-the-counter stool softeners as needed or MiraLAX if constipation is experienced.
- ❏ Eat small, frequent meals if you experience nausea.
- ❏ Rest with your head/back propped up if you experience nausea or difficulty breathing while lying down.
- ❏ Some providers recommend increasing your protein and electrolyte intake. Protein and electrolytes may help by increasing the osmolarity/concentration of your blood, which in turn helps to encourage fluid from the pelvic cavity/abdomen to move back into your bloodstream, which helps you feel less bloated.
- ❏ Stay hydrated by drinking plenty of fluids each day. Some women especially benefit from electrolyte-enhanced drinks such as coconut water, Nuun, or Gatorade.
- ❏ Consider increasing the protein in your diet with either protein-rich foods or protein powder:
  - ❏ For example, mix whey protein into your liquids – 20-25g (usually one scoop) up to four times a day as needed for improving bloating.
- ❏ Consider taking ibuprofen every 6-8 hours for the first few days to minimize or eliminate the need for narcotics.
- ❏ Get plenty of rest with your legs raised.
- ❏ Call your office if you experience:

- ❏ Excessive weight gain (more than three pounds in a 24-hour period).
- ❏ Severe abdominal pain.
- ❏ Nausea or vomiting where you cannot keep food or liquids down.
- ❏ Decreased urination with concentrated (dark in color) urine.
- ❏ Shortness of breath.
- ❏ Dizziness.
- ❏ Intense pelvic pain.

10

So I Have Frozen Eggs – What's Next? Understanding How to Use Them

Congratulations! Your egg freezing cycle is complete! Consider having a follow-up visit to review the cycle with your doctor. This is best done after you have recovered from the procedure so you can sit down and discuss what went well or as expected and what surprises (if any) there were. This is also a great time to discuss what changes would/could be made if you were to do another cycle and whether another cycle is right for you. Use this as a time to get any questions answered and to discuss next steps.

There are many factors that influence decision-making about another cycle. Some of these may include:

1. How many eggs you were able to freeze.
2. How well you tolerated the process and how quickly you recovered.
3. What your future family building goals are (how many kids you want to have).
4. How open you are to doing another cycle.
5. Remaining insurance benefit and amount of out of pocket costs.
6. How open you are to other family building options such as donor egg or adoption.
7. How long you plan to wait or how old you expect to be before trying to conceive.

Embryology

Now that you have frozen eggs, what would be the next steps if you wanted to use them? Whether you use a partner's sperm in the future or select a known or anonymous donor sperm source, you can return to the clinic that froze your egg(s) to review the thawing and fertilization process in hopes of embryo creation and eventual pregnancy.

After eggs are frozen on the day of the egg retrieval, they stay frozen until you are ready to fertilize them. Eggs are warmed in the embryology lab and fertilized. With fresh (not previously frozen) eggs, there are two types of fertilization methods. The first, called conventional insemination, is where eggs and sperm are placed in a dish together, and the second is ICSI (intracytoplasmic sperm injection), in which an embryologist selects the healthiest looking sperm and injects an individual sperm into the cytoplasm of each egg. When an egg has been frozen, the zona (shell around the egg) becomes a bit more difficult to penetrate, and the outer cumulus cells that are required for conventional insemination have been cleaned off, so ICSI is often chosen as the fertilization method. The day following, the embryologist can closely examine each egg to see if fertilization was successful. If it was, there should now be two nuclei, in what is now called an embryo.

From this point, embryos continue to grow in the embryology lab until day five or six of development. On average, 50% of the fertilized eggs will grow to the blastocyst stage. The attrition from a day two embryo to a day five to six embryo is highly variable. A blastocyst is a day five to six embryo of roughly 100-200 cells that has differentiated into the inner cell mass that would become the baby, as well as the trophectoderm that would become the placenta.

This is the stage that embryos can either be frozen using vitrification, biopsied for preimplantation genetic testing and then frozen, or transferred fresh into the uterus. Embryos that are frozen can be used at any point, and their chance of resulting in pregnancy does not decrease with time.

During the process of biopsying for preimplantation genetic testing (PGT), four to ten cells from the outer cell mass (the part that will become the placenta) are taken and sent to a genetic testing lab. The inner cell mass (the part that will become the baby) is not touched. The embryos themselves are stored at your clinic and typically do not leave your fertility center unless you arrange shipment or transfer to another storage facility.

The most common type of genetic testing is PGT-A (preimplantation genetic testing for aneuploidy). This testing has also been called chromosomal screening (CS) or preimplantation genetic screening (PGS). This is testing to see if the embryo has the correct number of chromosomes necessary to produce a healthy baby. This helps to select which embryo to transfer to the uterus – the one that will have the highest chance of resulting in a healthy pregnancy and live birth. It is an embryo selection tool that can help improve outcomes and reduce the risk of miscarriage.

In certain cases, other forms of preimplantation genetic testing (PGT) can be done to screen for specific disease-causing mutations or genetic structural rearrangements that may be inherited from one or both genetic parents. These are called PGT-M (PGT for monogenic/single gene disorders) and PGT-SR (PGT for chromosome structural rearrangements).

Just like eggs, embryos can be stored in an embryology lab or at a long-term storage facility until a patient is ready to try for pregnancy. When preparing for implantation, there are different hormonal medications and tests that will be recommended to prepare your uterus for an embryo transfer procedure and the possibility of implantation and pregnancy. This cycle is called a frozen embryo transfer (FET).

11
IVF With Embryo Banking for Fertility Preservation

When might it make sense to freeze embryos instead of eggs?
1. If you are partnered and ready to start trying or are wanting to save some for when you are ready.
2. If you are a single female or partnered with a woman and you are planning pregnancy with donor sperm, now or later.
3. If you have severely diminished ovarian reserve and you want to see if you can make a healthy embryo now.

Sometimes it makes sense to create and store embryos instead of eggs. This can be the case if you have already been trying for baby number one and you are seeking out fertility treatment. If you are struggling to conceive, it doesn't usually get easier for a subsequent pregnancy. You may want to also consider fertility preservation – saving embryos for future children – before undergoing your first embryo transfer and pregnancy.

Consider your family building goals. It is not uncommon for your goal to be, "We want two, maybe three kids someday, but we are just focusing on this first one." It is important to consider all options at this point, not only for fertility treatment for the immediate goal of pregnancy, but also fertility preservation for the children you hope to have in the future. Very few patients are focused on their overall family building goal up front. Most of us are, of course, focused on "How will I get pregnant with number one, ASAP?!!"

With the widespread use of the fast-freezing method called vitrification and preimplantation genetic testing of embryos for aneuploidy (PGT-A) making IVF success rates better than ever before, we are moving to a different era of family planning. While family planning has traditionally referred to birth control methods and access to abortion, the definition of family planning by the US Health Department is "the educational, comprehensive medical or social activities which enable individuals to determine freely the number and spacing of their children and to select the means by which this may be achieved." Just like a woman can proactively prevent pregnancy, she can also freeze her eggs or embryos in hopes of creating pregnancy in the future. We spend a lifetime learning and planning for our financial future – it is time to do the same for our fertility future.

Being a fertility patient when you are ready to have a baby is very traumatic. Every day, we see how frustrated women feel after spending a lifetime preventing pregnancy, only to find out that it can be harder to achieve pregnancy than they ever imagined. If you are already having difficulty conceiving, or if you are planning to wait until your mid to late 30s before attempting pregnancy, it's good to be aware that achieving pregnancy doesn't get easier with age. This changes the conversation from fertility treatment for immediate conception to include fertility preservation for possible subsequent pregnancies. While this does increase the time to pregnancy now, as patients may do more IVF cycles to save healthy (chromosomally 'normal') embryos for future children, it may help prevent infertility in the future. No one thinks achieving pregnancy will be difficult for them, but looking young and being healthy doesn't equal good fertility. Know the statistics, consider your family building goals, and learn about your options.

12
What Could Go Wrong? Hurdles to Egg Freezing

Although the majority of the time the egg freezing cycle will go smoothly, occasionally, unexpected challenges arise. The following list will help increase your awareness and hopefully decrease any anxiety. The "hurdles" are listed in the order they might occur:

❑ **Ovarian Cyst**: At the suppression check ultrasound, we are most commonly looking for ovaries at rest (no ovarian cysts), a low estradiol, and a thin endometrium (uterine lining). If any of these parameters are not met, it is possible that your cycle could be delayed. Most cysts are temporary and resolve on their own.

❑ **Inadequate Stimulation**: Some patients do not respond to ovarian stimulation medications (like FSH). If there is less follicular development than anticipated, the cycle may be canceled. If this occurs, your doctor will review the cycle with you and will likely determine a new plan in hopes of recruiting and developing more eggs in a new cycle.

❑ **Hyperstimulation**: A small percentage of women are extremely sensitive to ovulation induction medications. Rarely, it may be necessary to cancel the cycle and restart at a lower dose. Hyperstimulation can also occur after the egg retrieval and is called OHSS (ovarian hyperstimulation syndrome), which manifests primarily as abdominal bloating.

❑ **Unexpected Drop in Estradiol Level**: Typically, estradiol blood levels are measured during an egg freezing cycle. We expect the level to continue to rise during your cycle as the follicles grow.

❑ **Premature LH Surge/Progesterone Rise**: A few patients may experience a premature LH surge prior to achieving adequate follicular growth. If ovulation occurs prior to the egg retrieval procedure, no eggs will be retrieved during an egg retrieval procedure.

❑ **Low Number or Low Maturity of Eggs at Egg Retrieval**: Usually, the number of mature follicles (follicles >14mm) on the ultrasound on the day of the trigger is a reasonably close indication of the number of mature eggs that will be retrieved. Occasionally, the number of eggs retrieved is less than the expected yield. Often the science behind this can be confusing – counting follicles is our best guess at anticipated egg yield, but not every follicle produces an egg, and many other factors can contribute to varying egg counts at the time of retrieval.

❑ **No Eggs at Egg Retrieval**: This is extremely rare but can happen in some cases. The main causes are premature ovulation (ovulating prior to egg retrieval) or trigger injection failure.

Potential Future Hurdles When Using the Eggs:

❑ **Poor Fertilization of Eggs in the Future**: Standard fertilization rates are that 70-80% of mature eggs will fertilize, but there are large biological variabilities. In some cases, the percentage is much lower. Poor egg quality, poor sperm quality, and/or other factors may contribute to this occurrence.

❑ **No Fertilization**: Although this is extremely rare, it can happen that when eggs are thawed and fertilization is attempted, no eggs successfully fertilize.

❑ **No Embryo Creation**: Although eggs may thaw and fertilize successfully, there is still a risk that no day five to six embryos will result. This risk increases with low egg/embryo numbers, advanced maternal age, and poor sperm parameters.

❑ **Eggs That Do Not Survive the Thaw**: A certain percentage of eggs will not survive the thawing process. The chance that no eggs survive is very rare. Make sure to select a clinic with success in egg freezing and egg **thawing** and a clinic that has live births resulting from previously frozen eggs.

13
The 411 on Egg Freezing Medications and Giving Yourself Injections

Common Fertility Medications

Since not every egg results in a baby, the goal of ovarian stimulation in egg freezing and in IVF is to increase the number of eggs and follicles that mature in a given cycle over what would grow naturally in a cycle. The injectable medications used during a stimulation cycle are many of the same hormones that the body makes every month, just at higher doses to stimulate and mature multiple follicles. Many of these medications are like insulin and have to be injected (they cannot be taken in pill form). Here is a list of some common medications.

The Birth Control Pill

Using the birth control pill can help to organize the follicles to grow together and also helps with calendaring a cycle start. The birth control pill can help by preventing the body from recruiting a single dominant follicle to grow ahead of the rest (as occurs in the natural menstrual cycle). By preventing selection of a dominant/lead follicle, birth control pills (BCPs), also called oral contraceptive pills (OCPs), can promote more follicles to develop as a single cohort/group during a stimulation cycle. They are taken by mouth and are one of the only medications you don't have to inject! Only 'active' birth control pills are recommended, meaning that the week of placebo/sugar pills at the end of a pack of pills should not be taken as these pills would not prevent early follicular recruitment.

Follicle-Stimulating Hormone (FSH)

One of the most important medications used in an egg freezing cycle is follicle-stimulating hormone (FSH), which comes in many forms. FSH is used to recruit and grow multiple follicles and increase the number of eggs that develop in a cycle. In a natural menstrual cycle, the pituitary gland produces FSH hormone, which works at the ovaries to recruit and grow a follicle. During IVF, FSH is given in a higher dose than the brain makes naturally, with the goal of promoting multiple follicles to develop.

Luteinizing Hormone (LH)

Luteinizing hormone (LH) is also an important component in follicular growth. It can be added to a cycle as mini-hCG (a compounded medication) or other medications such as hMG (human menopausal gonadotropin).

Antagonist Medications

Antagonist medications work to prevent the body from releasing the eggs or ovulating early by preventing the body's LH surge.

Leuprolide Acetate

Lupron (leuprolide acetate) works in two ways. It can act similarly to an antagonist to suppress ovulation, and it does so by suppressing the body's own production of LH hormone from the pituitary gland. In this case, the Lupron is started prior to cycle start, often when a woman is still on a birth control pill. Lupron can also be used to stimulate follicular growth or trigger ovulation by stimulating the pituitary gland to release FSH/LH hormones. The effects of this medication vary widely, depending on when in the cycle this medication is administered.

The 'Trigger'

Once follicles are in the mature size range, your doctor will recommend "triggering" ovulation in preparation for the egg retrieval procedure. One common medication used is called human chorionic gonadotropin (hCG). HCG mimics an LH surge and helps eggs separate from the follicle wall and causes eggs to undergo final maturation. Typically, the egg retrieval will occur 35-36 hours after your trigger injection. Another common medication used to trigger final maturation of the eggs is Lupron. Lupron causes the brain to release LH. Your own LH is shorter acting, so this medication is sometimes used to decrease bloating following your procedure, especially in patients where a lot of eggs are anticipated.

The injectable medications used in an egg freezing cycle tend to be tolerated very well. The most common symptom seen is injection site irritation such as redness, itching, bruising, or bleeding. If you hit a small vessel, it causes a little bruising, and if you hit a small nerve, it hurts more. Neither causes the medication not to work. If you get a little bleeding following an injection, apply pressure like you would if you had your blood drawn to help prevent bruising. If it hurts more in a certain area, just avoid that area in the future.

Medication doses and protocols can vary by practice, by patient, and by doctor – and from cycle to cycle. This information is intended to educate and be a guide, but it is not medical advice. Be sure to ask your care team if you have questions or concerns about your recommended protocol.

Injection Tips!

Prior to an egg freezing cycle, it is a good idea to set aside some time to review your cycle calendar, review any outstanding requirements, review and sign necessary consent forms, ask any remaining questions you may have, and review tips and injection training materials. Sometimes a "nurse visit" or "injection training" appointment or class is offered or available at your clinic.

Watching an injection administration video (typically available online or through your clinic or pharmacy) can also make the whole process less intimidating. An instructional video can help calm some of the injection nerves and allow you to figure out what questions you may have. It also seems to help patients retain more information during the in person visit and relieve some initial nerves. Feeling confident in this skill (even though it's a little scary) is important, as soon you will be doing it on your own.

If you are planning a special visit with your doctor's office to review the injections, then reviewing consent forms prior to that visit can be beneficial in making sure you fully understand the process and risks, and to help gather any remaining questions you may have. Doing this ahead of time can make the first injections a little less stressful. There are a lot of wonderful video resources that can be accessed for free online or as part of your clinic's consenting process. Ask your clinic or pharmacy for resources and recommendations if needed.

The first couple of injections will likely feel a little overwhelming and weird, but patients usually tolerate fertility injections and medications pretty well. The injections usually aren't very painful, but icing the area first or trying a numbing patch (ask your nurse!) prior to injecting may help those with a fear of needles or pain with injections.

You really can't mess it up! Insert the full length of the needle into the skin at a 90 degree angle for intramuscular (in the muscle) injections and a 45 to 90 degree angle for subcutaneous (in the skin) injections. Don't panic if you see a little drop of blood, medication coming out, or a bruise after an injection. As mentioned above, sometimes you hit a little blood vessel that you can't see, and it bruises a little. Sometimes you hit a little nerve, and it hurts or burns a little. If this happens, you could avoid that area on your skin in the future.

Other calming strategies that some patients find helpful are deep breathing before and after, lying down to give the injection, eating or drinking some water first, or having a friend or partner administer the injections. You've got this!

14

Common Questions and Mistakes

Common Questions

"Does an egg freezing cycle hurt my future fertility potential?"

This is one of the most common questions that patients have, and it's an important one to understand. There is no evidence that egg freezing has a negative impact on future fertility. An ovarian stimulation cycle does not decrease the overall egg supply but utilizes eggs in a cycle that would otherwise be lost that month. During each cycle, there are a certain number of potential eggs (or antral follicles) available. If unused, these eggs simply die off. An egg freezing cycle rescues this group of follicles that would otherwise be lost or unused that month, meaning it does not reduce the number of eggs you may have remaining in your ovaries for your future fertility.

"How many eggs do I need to freeze?"

This is a complicated question. Each person and scenario varies widely. How many children do you want? How long do you intend to wait until you start trying to conceive? How old will you be at the time of the egg retrieval? Age is the largest contributor to success rates, so it is often recommended that women who are older at the time of freezing eggs freeze a larger number of eggs for use in the future – knowing that the percentage of good eggs declines with advancing age. That being said, the number of eggs that you can collect in a single cycle typically decreases with advancing age as well, making this a less efficient process. Having an understanding of the average attrition rates from egg to embryo at your age can help you make an educated decision about how many eggs you may want to save for future use. It is important to remember that these numbers are all statistics and that many other factors impact these numbers/rates, some of which are very poorly understood. There are many biological differences that create variability in success rates.

On average, 80% of mature eggs will fertilize. From the eggs that fertilize, an average of 50% will reach the blastocyst stage of embryo development. This is the stage in which freezing, transferring fresh to the uterus, or preimplantation genetic testing can occur. For females, at the age of 35, roughly 50% of tested embryos will be chromosomally suitable for transfer (genetically normal).

In summary, if ten mature eggs are frozen at an age less than 35, on average, eight eggs would fertilize, four would reach the blastocyst stage, and two would be chromosomally 'normal' embryos. The average live birth rate can be as high as a 60-70% chance per euploid embryo (having the correct number of chromosomes based on genetic testing), but this varies widely from clinic to clinic. This example can help tailor how many mature eggs you may want based on your age. These averages are to be used as a guide, and it is not uncommon for patients to exceed the average or to feel disappointment if these numbers are not met. There are many factors that impact success when using frozen eggs, and unfortunately, there are no guarantees in the future, so consider trying to save more than you think you will need.

Disclaimer: The above information is based on averages from 2020 data. It is important to note that each clinic and lab does vary and that these values may change with time.

"How can I make the process easier?"
Keeping your schedule lighter and more open and flexible during the time of stimulation is helpful in reducing the burden that the process can cause on your life. Understand that there are many biological variabilities that affect the timing of an egg freezing cycle and that your follicles may not follow the calendar you have for them. It is important to get them out at just the right time, and they may not be ready on the day you think they should be. Finding a clinic and team that you feel comfortable with so you can trust your nurse and your doctor also makes the process easier. Consider also having the support

of a friend or partner or someone in your personal life that you can share the journey with. And finally, just by reading this and educating yourself, you are empowering yourself and making the process easier. The more you understand, the less scary it feels.

Building in ways to relieve stress can also help. Some patients like acupuncture, others find a support group or talk with their counselor, read a book, go to yoga, or go for a walk. Finding a friend, partner, or confidant can make a huge difference. Let your care team know if you have questions and how they can help support you best.

"What vitamins or supplements can I take when preparing for egg freezing?"

This is one of the most common questions patients ask in preparation for their egg freezing cycle. (See Chapter Six for details on preparing for your egg freezing cycle for a list of popular supplements). In general, you should consider prenatal vitamins, CoQ10, and vitamin D. But this list may change and can differ depending on patient needs and diagnoses. Talk with your doctor about what vitamins/supplements might be right for you. Also, focus on a healthy diet, eliminate alcohol/smoking, minimize caffeine, and get adequate sleep.

Common Mistakes

It is easy to feel overwhelmed if you make a mistake. Most of the time, there is an easy fix or adjustment that can be made. Some mistakes are quite common – because they're so easy to do! By sharing this list, we hope to prevent these bumps in the road from happening to you:

- ❏ **Don't forget to stop your birth control pill.** Often, a specific number of days on birth control pills is recommended, meaning that some patients are on more or less than the 21 days that come in a typical pack of pills. If it is recommended for you to take the pill, the intention is only to have you take the "active pills" (no placebo/sugar pills) and to follow your calendar exactly – stopping when indicated on the calendar, even if there are active pills remaining in the pack. Additionally, if your pack runs out of active pills and your calendar recommends continuing, request a refill from your pharmacy so you can continue taking active pills only. Often, patients are on autopilot and just continue taking the pill to finish the pill pack, but be mindful of the day that you have been instructed to stop.

❏ **Don't take the placebo pills.** The last week of birth control pills in a standard pack are usually a different color. These are the placebo/sugar pills and should not be taken unless specifically directed.

❏ **Pay attention to what pharmacy you need to order from.** Egg freezing medications typically come from specialty fertility pharmacies that are mail order. If you have insurance coverage for fertility medications, contact your insurance directly and ask which specialty fertility pharmacy they prefer you to use. Let your care team know so that your prescription can be submitted. If you do not have insurance coverage or are paying out of pocket, let your nurse coordinator know so they can help you find the lowest 'cash' pay options or provide a list of available pharmacies to choose from.

❏ **Get your medications a couple days early.** It is typically recommended that you get your medications at least a couple of days ahead of your estimated stimulation start date. You don't want a shipping complication to cause stress or possibly delay your stimulation start.

❏ **Don't forget to open the box and refrigerate medications.** Some of the medications need to be refrigerated, so be sure to examine your medication shipment when it arrives and place refrigerated items directly in the refrigerator (do NOT freeze).

❏ **Don't throw away partially empty vials.** These medications are very expensive, so keep your FSH cartridges/pens in the refrigerator after you take your dose.

The FSH cartridges are overfilled and have small amounts of 'extra' medication that can be used as needed (even if it looks empty!). If you end up needing more medications toward the end of your cycle, it is possible to combine the small remainders in the seemingly almost empty cartridges/pens to hopefully help save a little of the medication cost.

❑ **Know your administration tool**. There are many online resources that provide educational videos on how to administer the injectable ovarian stimulation medications. These medications can be tricky, and mistakes and confusion are not uncommon. Contact your nurse coordinator with questions to help clarify confusion and minimize mistakes during your egg freezing cycle.

❑ **Know how to get urgent questions answered**. Know how to get your questions answered both during and after office hours. Some practices have a special number or email for patients that need help after the office is closed. Knowing how to get help if you need it can prevent anxiety should any urgent need arise.

15
Side Effects of Egg Freezing

Most people tolerate the egg freezing cycle well, but knowing the side effects and what you can do to treat or avoid them can help you feel more prepared. If you do experience discomfort, the most common symptoms that are seen during an egg freezing stimulation cycle include headaches, fatigue, and bloating.

Headaches

Headaches are often caused by the fluctuating levels of estrogen in your body during an egg freezing cycle. They tend to be the worst right at the beginning of the cycle (when estrogen levels are low) and improve as the follicles grow and produce estrogen. Tylenol and other over-the-counter headache medications are safe to use for headaches, and remember that rest and hydration can also help.

Fatigue

Your body is working hard during an egg freezing cycle and making estrogen, which can cause fatigue. This is also a very busy time balancing your everyday life with all the office visits, ultrasounds, and blood draws. To minimize stress and fatigue, build extra time into your schedule to make it to appointments and to rest if needed.

Bloating

Bloating is one of the most common symptoms that women experience and is due to the increased size of the ovaries. During an egg freezing cycle, the goal is more than one follicle (egg) to grow. Often, more follicles mean more eggs, but it can also mean more bloating. With this can come pelvic discomfort and fluid retention as well as temporary weight gain due to increased fluid volume and increased ovarian size. It can start at any time during the stimulation cycle, but often is most noticeable toward the end. It can also continue up until one to two weeks after the egg retrieval procedure. Not everyone experiences bloating. Most women experience just mild bloating, but some women experience a more intense form of bloating and even rarely OHSS (ovarian hyperstimulation syndrome). Some experience constipation and/or nausea associated with the bloating.

Ovarian Hyperstimulation Syndrome (OHSS)

Ovarian hyperstimulation syndrome (OHSS) is a rare complication of egg freezing more common at younger ages and higher AMH levels, where the bloating is much more severe. If you experience more severe symptoms, make sure to let your clinical team know so that you can be monitored closely. The best way to prevent severe bloating is to start at a lower dose of egg freezing medications or use a Lupron trigger at the end of the cycle. Even if all these things are done, some women still experience OHSS – everyone is different! (Please refer to Chapter 9 for more information about recovery from the egg freezing cycle and tips for bloating).

Vaginal Discharge

Some patients experience increased vaginal discharge/cervical mucus that is commonly associated with ovulation. This is due to rising estrogen blood levels during the cycle. Do not be alarmed – this is normal.

Breast Tenderness

Breast tenderness or other PMS-like symptoms can be common due to higher than normal estrogen and progesterone blood levels during the cycle.

Injection Site Irritation

Skin irritation, redness, itching around the injection site, and bruising are all very commonly associated with giving injections. While uncomfortable, these are very normal and will go away. Icing the area after an injection may help prevent pain while holding pressure following the injection can decrease bruising.

Emotional Changes

Some fertility drugs are known to contribute to irritability and 'moodiness,' but in general, this is not typically seen with egg freezing medications. Most women continue to work and function normally during the egg freezing process, but it is important to note that everyone's experience is slightly different.

Weight Gain

While some women report an increase in weight during the egg freezing cycle, this usually completely resolves, and women return to their normal body weight by the time they get their next menstrual cycle 7-10 days after their egg retrieval. This weight gain is often due to bloating from the growth of the ovary and fluid retention that occurs with ovarian stimulation.

Accidental Pregnancy

This is a theoretical risk, but it is the reason for the recommendation to avoid unprotected intercourse during the stimulation cycle.

16

Choosing a Clinic

If you want to start the process of fertility preservation, your first and sometimes most daunting task is to choose a clinic. Not every fertility clinic is created equal. Here is what you should know:

1. **The egg freeze.** The embryology piece of egg freezing is a big deal. The process of vitrification (fast freeze method) is what makes egg freezing successful. The egg is the largest cell in the human body, and it is fragile. Handling it requires TLC from someone with a lot of technical expertise. In fact, egg freezing was considered experimental by the American Society of Reproductive Medicine (ASRM) until 2012. To date, there are still only thousands of babies born from previously frozen eggs in the US. It is important that the clinic and embryology lab has a long history of freezing and thawing eggs and has pregnancy data on outcomes from frozen eggs. It is okay to ask who will be freezing your eggs, how much experience they have, and how many live births have occurred from frozen eggs at that clinic. These are just some of the things to consider, and since these are your potential future children, it's a really big deal.

2. **The future thaw.** Many clinics freeze eggs, but fewer have as much experience in successfully warming the eggs and creating embryos that result in successful pregnancies. It can be done with expert technical expertise and still not be successful, so it's important to trust that you are in the best hands. Reproductive biology is an imperfect process (including in nature), and there is a lot of attrition that occurs between warming (thawing) the egg and making an embryo. This means that potentially not all the eggs will survive the thawing process, not all of the eggs that survive the thaw will successfully fertilize with sperm, not all fertilized eggs will become a viable embryo, not all embryos

will be genetically compatible with life, and not all of the embryos (fertilized eggs) will become a baby when transferred into the uterus (even when genetic testing has been done). When you are considering egg freezing, talk to your doctor about how many eggs you should freeze. The eggs are the oldest cells in your body, and as you age, so do your eggs. The older you are, the more eggs you should freeze in order to give yourself the highest chance of success in the future (due to declining egg quality with age). The success rate per embryo is driven by the age at which the eggs were frozen. And, as you know, freezing your eggs is never a guarantee of a baby, so make sure you have realistic expectations about how they can be used in the future.

3. **Find a good-fit clinic where you are comfortable.** In addition to technical expertise, it is also important to find a good-fit clinic and doctor where you feel comfortable and confident with your clinical team. The egg freezing process is no walk in the park, but feeling well taken care of makes a huge difference. If you decide to move forward to freezing your eggs, you will have quite a few appointments, and you will have to walk in, take off your pants, and be okay with it. While a medical clinic is not a spa, feeling comfortable in your surroundings and having all your questions answered will have a lot to do with how you'll feel throughout the process.

4. **Buddy up!** Know who is going to be walking with you through the egg-freezing process. Who will you see for most of your appointments? Will the physician be doing your ultrasounds or will it be an ultrasound tech? Who will be communicating next steps to you? You also want to ask how you will get your questions answered. Seeing the same people who know you and know your story can make the process a more positive one and will help make the experience of egg freezing a little easier.

5. **Figure out the finances**. Egg freezing is expensive and often an out of pocket cost, meaning not covered by insurance. Often finances are the limiting factor when considering preserving fertility. Unfortunately, cheaper does not equal better, and you don't want suboptimal results in order to save a little bit of money. Certainly, egg freezing is expensive and a big decision, but don't let cost be your number-one determinant.

6. **Know what your egg storage plan is**. Some clinics plan to keep your eggs at their facility, while others send the eggs off site to a "long-term" storage facility. There are advantages and disadvantages to both options. Things to consider include safety of moving eggs, benefits of thawing and using eggs at the clinic where they were frozen, and potential cost savings of longer term storage sites.

Now that you know the basics of choosing a clinic, your next step is to make an appointment with the clinic you think is the best fit for you. Go to your appointment, learn about your fertility, and ask about what that clinic has to offer. Make sure the above criteria are met and that you feel comfortable with the provider, the place, and the process, and then go for it. If something doesn't feel right, it's always okay to meet with another provider or get another opinion. Egg freezing is empowering and life changing, but it's also hard and extremely personal, and you want to make sure that you have a supportive team on your side.

17

The Finances of Egg Freezing

There are a lot of factors that go into deciding to freeze your eggs, but a big one of these is cost. We are encouraged from a young age to plan and invest for our financial futures, but not many people encourage you to proactively plan for your future family. Egg freezing is an investment in your future fertility, and like any investment, it is important to educate yourself about costs as you consider the process.

Medical care is expensive, and egg freezing is no exception. The biggest difference is that this is often an out of pocket cost not covered by insurance. It is much easier to freeze your eggs if it is a covered benefit by your employer as it eliminates the huge stress of figuring out how you are going to pay for it. When it is an out of pocket cost, remember that cheaper doesn't equal better. Make sure to really understand the embryology lab and their statistics on successful live births from frozen eggs (see Chapter 16 on choosing a clinic). Ironically, often by the time you can afford to pay for egg freezing, you have aged out of the window where it is most successful.

It is important to truly understand the total costs of egg freezing, as sometimes the costs quoted by clinics don't include things that you ultimately need as part of the process, such as medications or the cost of yearly storage. Educate yourself on the different costs of egg freezing and which costs are associated with each step. The graph below gives some examples of cost categories.

Medication:
> Birth control pills
> Simulation medication
> Trigger medication

Clinic fees:
    Ultrasounds
    Blood work
Egg Retrieval Procedure costs
    Anesthesia costs

Embryology costs:
    Oocyte identification
Oocyte vitrification (freezing)

Storage fee per year

TOTAL COST

Let's break down the process by each step. One of the first (and sometimes biggest) costs are the egg freezing medications. Stimulation medications are very specialized and expensive. Prices vary between pharmacies and vary by protocol and medication dose (typically determined by ovarian reserve values). If your medication is covered by insurance, that's a huge win, but pay attention – you may need to order your medications from a specific pharmacy in order to have your insurance cover them. Also of note, if you are paying cash, you can often get a discounted rate (cash pay price) from your pharmacy, which is less than they would bill to insurance – so don't be afraid to ask and to shop around.

Clinic costs are the next big piece of egg freezing, and they can vary widely. Clinic costs include things such as ultrasounds and blood work that are done during your cycle to watch your follicles grow. Also included in the clinic cost is the egg aspiration procedure (retrieval), which often includes a surgical facility fee and anesthesia cost. These are big expenses that you often don't consider if you're having a medical procedure that's covered by insurance. Did you know that even the specialized disposable needle used to collect your eggs is quite expensive?

The next costs are the embryology services related to identifying the eggs from the follicular fluid at the time of egg retrieval and the process of freezing them. It is also important to consider the cost of storing your eggs until you are ready to use them. This is called the storage fee and can also vary widely. The eggs are kept in highly regulated tanks of liquid nitrogen that require lots of checking and many back up processes in order to keep them as safe as possible. Moving your eggs to a long-term storage facility can be less expensive, especially if you don't plan to use them for many years.

So when does freezing eggs become cost effective? You really need a crystal ball to tell you if you are going to meet someone and have no difficulty conceiving your ideal family. But since that isn't possible, egg freezing allows you to save eggs in case you aren't able to conceive naturally when you are ready in the future. There have been several studies looking at when egg freezing becomes cost effective, and in general, if a woman plans to delay childbearing until age 40, then egg freezing before the age of 38 lowers the cost to obtain a live birth.[1] But this does not mean you should wait until you're 38 to freeze your eggs, if possible, and it also does not mean that if you are over 38 and well counseled that egg freezing is not for you. It is important to figure out when/if it is right for you, and this varies widely based on age, current relationship factors, insurance benefit, ability to pay for it, and overall family building goals. So many factors go into this type of decision – it is important to have this conversation with a provider you trust.

[1]Devine K, Mumford SL, Goldman KN, et al. Baby budgeting: oocyte cryopreservation in women delaying reproduction can reduce cost per live birth. Fertil Steril 2015;103:1446-53.

18
Chances of Success Using Frozen Eggs

There are many factors that affect egg freezing success rates and make it tricky to understand. The introduction of vitrification (a fast-freezing method) has changed the way we think about eggs and success rates. In fact, this was the factor that made egg freezing much more successful and mainstream. Yet there are still many biological inefficiencies of egg freezing, and it can take many frozen eggs to make an embryo and eventually a baby.

The below graph interprets data from a study that was published by a group at Harvard in *Human Reproduction*, a leading reproductive medical journal, in 2017. It is currently some of the best data we have when counseling women about their chance of success based on age and number of eggs frozen. The study includes data from 520 healthy women undergoing fertility treatment. It is an excellent tool to help you understand how the chances of conception change with age and how saving more eggs improves your chance of a successful pregnancy in the future. One thing that all studies show is that the younger a woman is when she freezes her eggs, the better the chance those eggs will lead to a healthy baby. This is because the younger a woman's eggs, the more likely they will lead to genetically normal embryos (higher **quality**), and when a woman is younger, she is more likely to respond better to the stimulation process and produce more eggs in a single cycle (higher **quantity**). For example, this predicts that a woman under the age of 35 who freezes 10-20 eggs will have between a 70-90% chance of at least one live birth if the eggs were used in the future.

Everyone processes and uses this data a little differently. Sometimes a woman at 39 will decide not to freeze her eggs because freezing 10 eggs only gives her a 40% chance of a baby in the future. This woman may decide that she would rather adopt or use donor eggs if not able to conceive when ready. Or she may decide to try to conceive earlier than planned, even if it involves donor sperm. Another woman may decide that freezing 10 eggs at age 42 is totally worth it for her, even if it only gives her a 20% chance of a baby. Everyone's path is different, and as long as you have realistic expectations and an understanding of the success rates, it is not wrong to undergo egg freezing, even if your chances are lower than you would like them to be. We see egg freezing as one more possible option of family planning.

Assisted reproductive technology (ART) with egg freezing can be an amazing tool to allow women the possibility to conceive later in their reproductive life, but remember, it is not an insurance policy. It is not always successful. The eggs you save do NOT have a 100% chance of success in the future. Even though you feel and look young, many of the eggs will not have a normal chromosome count. It is therefore very important to thoroughly understand your chances of success and plan accordingly.

Likelihood that a woman will have at least one live birth at a given age and number of mature oocytes retrieved[1]

AGE	10 Eggs	20 Eggs
≤35	69%	90%
36-37	50-60%	75-84%
38-39	39-45%	63-69%
40	30%	51%
41-42	20-25%	37-44%
43-44	8-14%	15-25%

[1]Adapted from Goldman RH, Racowsky C, Farland LV, Munné S, Ribustello L, Fox JH. Predicting the likelihood of live birth for elective oocyte cryopreservation: a counseling tool for physicians and patients. Hum Reprod 2017;32:853-9.
https://doi.org/10.1093/humrep/dex008

19

The Quick and Dirty Summary

The basics of egg freezing:

❏ Oocyte cryopreservation, the scientific name for egg freezing, is a technique that allows women to preserve their eggs (on ice!) until they are ready to conceive. Egg freezing can also be used to preserve fertility for women who may be faced with new medical diagnoses where treatment can compromise future fertility potential.

❏ By reading this information, you are taking the first step to considering fertility preservation, learning more about your options, educating yourself, and becoming an advocate for your own fertility!

❏ According to the ASRM (American Society for Reproductive Medicine), one out of seven couples have trouble conceiving. Fertility preservation can help reduce the risk of infertility by empowering patients to plan for their future earlier on.

❏ Fertility preservation usually begins with a consultation at a fertility center, followed by a fertility evaluation to determine the potential success and efficiency of freezing eggs. A typical consultation reviews your health history, your plans for fertility testing, and what you can expect during the egg freezing process. Testing can involve an ultrasound as well as blood tests that give an idea about the quality and quantity of your egg supply or "ovarian reserve." The timing of the fertility testing is dependent on your menstrual cycle, so it may take up to a month for you to get those tests completed. Your provider will review the test results with you, counsel you about your personal chances for success, and make recommendations for a personalized treatment regimen.

❏ The stimulation phase of IVF (egg freezing) often involves two to three injections a day ranging from nine to fourteen days, depending on how your ovaries respond to the hormonal medications. The medications are used to stimulate more follicles to grow. Growth is monitored using vaginal ultrasound and estrogen blood levels. The eggs are then retrieved from the follicles and frozen for later use.

❏ When you are ready to conceive, your frozen eggs can be thawed and fertilized with sperm (partner or donor), and embryos can be created and placed in the uterus to cause pregnancy.

❏ While there are no guarantees on the success of the eggs when warmed, this is a great option for many to preserve their current fertility potential in hopes of combating the decline in egg quality and quantity that occurs with age.

❏ Life is complicated, with a range of stressors including relationships, finances, careers, families, and more – sometimes freezing eggs can help relieve some of the pressure and empower women to take charge of their body and future.

Summary of what your testing will typically include:

❏ **FSH and Estradiol**: Blood tests that are drawn on cycle day two or three of your menstrual cycle that primarily evaluate the quality of your egg supply. FSH is produced by your pituitary gland and helps to stimulate the ovaries to recruit and develop a follicle during the menstrual cycle. If the FSH level gets high (>10), it gives an idea that the egg quality may be diminished as your brain is working too hard to get the ovaries to respond in order to ovulate. According to ASRM, an elevated FSH level indicates that your chances for pregnancy may be lower than routinely expected for your age, especially if you are 35 or older.

❏ **AMH (Anti-Müllerian Hormone)**: This can be drawn on any day of the cycle and primarily evaluates the quantity of the egg supply. AMH is produced by other cells in the ovaries and gives us an idea of the quantity of the remaining egg supply.

❏ **Transsvaginal Ultrasound**: This is often completed at your new patient visit. An antral follicle count is done as another way to look at potential egg supply in addition to being a general fertility and gynecologic assessment of the anatomy of the ovaries and uterus.

❏ **Virologies (HIV, HepB Ab, HepB Ag, Hep C)**: These are often required prior to egg freezing.

❏ **TSH (Thyroid-Stimulating Hormone)**: A thyroid function test can be done before the egg freeze cycle to prevent possible complications with anesthesia and assess general health.

These lab tests – particularly the FSH, estradiol, and AMH – give us an idea of how you may respond to the injectable fertility medications. The AMH and FSH levels along with information gathered in a transvaginal ultrasound (counting resting follicles on the ovaries) as well as factors such as age and previous cycles allow your fertility provider to select a medication protocol and dose for your egg freezing cycle.

What can you do to get ahead of your fertility?

1. **Ask your doctor for fertility testing at your yearly well woman visit.** This is an AMH level and can be followed over time as a little window into your fertility. It doesn't tell you if it will be hard to achieve pregnancy, but it does tell you if you have eggs left. Every woman is different, and you don't want to find out when it is too late that you are out of eggs.

2. **Take care of your health.** Minimize alcohol and eliminate marijuana, minimize reproductive toxins in your life, and protect yourself from sexually transmitted infections that can cause infertility.

3. **Talk to a fertility specialist and learn about your options.** Think about preserving your fertility with egg freezing or embryo freezing and whether it's right for you.

What can you do when you are in the middle of egg freezing treatment?

1. **Know your fertility.** Understand how age and ovarian reserve affect your chances of conceiving in the future.
2. **Define your overall family building goal.** Consider saving more eggs if you desire more than one child in order to have a greater chance of meeting your goal.
3. **Make a plan.** Talk to your fertility specialist and make a treatment plan that is right for you to meet your family building goal. This could involve saving eggs or embryos for future pregnancy attempts.
4. **Don't compare.** Every patient is different, and no plan is the same, and that is okay. Everyone's resources – physical, emotional, and financial – are limited in different ways. Allow yourself to feel confident in yourself, your doctor, and your plan for your future family.

Choosing a clinic:

1. See what's out there in your area. Is there a reputable clinic in your area? Read reviews, ask friends for referrals, and look at the information on the clinic's website.
2. Make sure that the doctor you choose is board certified in reproductive endocrinology and infertility (REI); this means they are fellowship trained and have passed the strictest examinations in the field.
3. Ask about the embryology lab and where the eggs will be collected and stored.
4. Inquire about their live birth rates from frozen eggs (it is easy to freeze eggs, but thawing eggs can have highly variable success rates).
5. Ask who you will be seeing during the cycle and what is the best way to communicate with your doctor or your team if you have questions. (See Chapter 16 for more information on how to choose a clinic).

Tips for success during the egg freezing process:
1. **Take care of yourself.** Make sure you get enough sleep, especially when your ovaries are being stimulated. Minimize stress. Prioritizing your cycle by limiting social and work obligations can help make the process a little easier. Fertility preservation is a time-consuming process. The length of time on injections and dates that you will need to be in and out of the office vary from person to person and with each cycle. It is difficult to predict the outcome ahead of time, and this can be frustrating.
2. **Eliminate toxins.** Take care of yourself, and your eggs will appreciate it! Eat right – lots of organic fruits and vegetables – and minimize or eliminate processed foods. Minimize or eliminate alcohol and caffeine, and eliminate tobacco and marijuana. Make your health your top priority! Consider limiting BPA exposure and other toxins frequently seen in food storage containers, cleaning supplies, and beauty products.
3. **Take your vitamins.** Take a multivitamin or a prenatal vitamin that includes folate or folic acid. Also consider adding CoQ10/ubiquinol (400mcg/day), omega-3 fatty acids, and vitamin D (minimum 800IU).
4. **Exercise, but in moderation.** During the stimulation process, it is typically recommended to avoid vigorous exercise the week prior and the week following your egg retrieval. Walking is always okay – some fresh air and movement is good for you – but limit or eliminate high impact exercise during treatment.
5. **Educate yourself.** Knowledge is power. It is important to know that freezing eggs doesn't ever guarantee you a baby in the future. The success rates and number of eggs retrieved vary widely by patient. When the egg supply is low or with advancing age, often patients will need to consider doing

several cycles compared to someone who has a higher egg supply.

Fertility preservation with egg freezing is an empowering option for women who are not ready to start their family. The field has seen tremendous success and many advances in the last ten years, but fertility preservation should be viewed as an option or opportunity, not a guarantee of fertility in the future. Wishing you healthy eggs and future fertility!

    – Dr. Julie Lamb and Nurse Emily Gray

Glossary of Terms and Acronyms

AFC (Antral Follicle Count): A subjective count of resting follicles on each ovary done with pelvic ultrasound.

AMH (Anti-Müllerian Hormone): A hormone produced by supporting cells around the eggs in the ovaries that will be available that month.

Aneuploid: A term used to refer to an embryo that does not have the correct number of chromosomes considered necessary to produce a healthy baby.

ART (Assisted Reproductive Technology): Advanced fertility treatment including in vitro fertilization, egg freezing, donor egg, and embryo transfer cycles.

ASRM (American Society of Reproductive Medicine): Professional society of reproductive endocrinologists that publishes patient education materials and hosts the educational website reproductivefacts.org.

BCPs (Birth Control Pills): Also known as oral contraceptive pills (OCPs). Fertility preservation cycles sometimes start with birth control pills for a time leading up to the injection or stimulation phase. The intention of the pill is not to prevent pregnancy but to briefly suppress the ovaries to organize the follicles and prevent a dominant follicle from coming forward – thus producing a cohort of follicles with similar sizes.

Chromosomal Screening or Preimplantation Genetic Screening (CS or PGS): The most common type of genetic testing is PGT-A (preimplantation genetic testing for aneuploidy). This testing has also been called chromosomal screening (CS) or preimplantation genetic screening (PGS). This testing is done on the embryo (not the egg) to evaluate if it has the correct number of chromosomes necessary to produce a healthy baby. This can help select which embryo to transfer to the uterus to have the highest chance of resulting in a healthy pregnancy and live birth. It is an embryo selection tool that can help improve outcomes and reduce the risk of miscarriage. It involves a biopsy on day five or six of embryo development from the trophectoderm (portion that would become the placenta) and is sent to an outside lab for testing.

DOR (Diminished Ovarian Reserve): A lower ovarian reserve supply, often quantified by a FSH (follicle-stimulating hormone) value >10 mIU/mL and/or an AMH (Anti-Müllerian Hormone) <1.0 ng/mL. A high FSH and low AMH value does not mean you cannot conceive if you were trying to get pregnant; however, it may predict a lower response to the stimulation process.

EEF (Elective Egg Freezing): The first half of IVF, in which a woman grows follicles and mature eggs that can be collected from her ovary, frozen, and saved for later use.

ER (Egg Retrieval): The egg (oocyte) retrieval is a procedure in which eggs are removed from the ovaries at the conclusion of ovarian stimulation.

ET (Embryo Transfer): An embryo can be transferred into the uterus through a thin/flexible catheter through the cervix when ready to conceive.

Euploid: Referring to an embryo whose genetic testing showed the correct number of chromosomes necessary to produce a healthy baby.

E2 (Estrogen or Estradiol): A hormone produced by developing follicles that often guide decisions during an egg freezing cycle.

FET (Frozen Embryo Transfer): Eggs can be made into embryos, and, like eggs, embryos can be stored in an embryology lab or long-term storage facility for later use. When you are preparing for implantation and pregnancy, there are protocols of different hormonal medications that prepare your uterus for an embryo transfer procedure and pregnancy. Often, this entire process can be referred to as an FET. An embryo can be warmed on the day of an embryo transfer procedure – this is called a frozen embryo transfer.

Follicle: A fluid-filled sac in the ovary that likely contains an egg. A follicle can be measured on ultrasound.

Follicular Phase: The first half of the menstrual cycle in which an egg grows and matures within a follicle, causing the endometrial lining to grow and thicken. The follicular phase ends when ovulation occurs.

FSH (Follicle-Stimulating Hormone): A hormone secreted from the pituitary gland that encourages a follicle to grow and mature in the first half of the menstrual cycle (the follicular phase). One of the most important medications used in a fertility preservation cycle. When taken as a medication, it is injected (it cannot be taken by mouth). There are many different brand names for this medication. FSH is used to recruit and grow multiple follicles and increase the number of eggs that develop in a cycle. In a natural menstrual cycle, the pituitary gland produces FSH hormone, which works on the ovaries to recruit and grow a follicle. During ovarian stimulation, FSH is given in a higher dose than the brain makes with the goal of promoting multiple follicles to develop.

hCG (Human Chorionic Gonadotropin): hCG hormone is produced by the placenta after implantation. hCG is the hormone of pregnancy that is tested in a pregnancy test. hCG can also be a hormone given to mature the follicles (in low doses) or at the time of "trigger" to induce final oocyte maturation (high dose).

hMG (Human Menopausal Gonadotropin): hMG is a common source of hormones used in IVF treatments, a mixture of the two gonadotropins purified from the urine of postmenopausal women.

ICSI (Intracytoplasmic Sperm Injection): ICSI is a method of fertilization in which an embryologist selects a single sperm and injects it into the cytoplasm of each egg.

IVF (In Vitro Fertilization): IVF is the process of growing follicles, collecting the eggs, fertilizing them, and creating embryos. With egg freezing, the eggs are cryopreserved prior to fertilization, but the process of growing follicles and maturing the eggs inside the body is the same. IVF is a "high tech" fertility treatment option that involves ovarian stimulation using injectable hormonal medications to promote the growth of more follicles (fluid-filled sacs in the ovary that likely contain an egg) to mature during one cycle than would normally occur during a natural cycle alone.

LH (Luteinizing Hormone): LH is an important hormone in follicular growth. A surge of LH hormone during a natural menstrual cycle causes ovulation (the release of the egg from the follicle) to occur.

Luteal Phase: The second half of the menstrual cycle – beginning with ovulation and lasting until the start of the following menses.

Menstrual Cycle: The menstrual cycle is counted from the first day of a period (full flow bleeding before 9 pm, not including spotting) to the first day of the subsequent period. The menstrual cycle consists of the follicular and luteal phases and typically lasts an average of 28 days.

OCPs (Oral Contraceptive Pills): OCPS are birth control pills. The IVF or egg freezing stimulation cycle can start with birth control pills for the time leading up to the injection phase. The intention of the pill is not to prevent pregnancy, but to briefly suppress the ovaries to organize the follicles and prevent a dominant one from coming forward, thus producing a cohort of follicles with similar sizes.

OHSS (Ovarian Hyperstimulation Syndrome): A small percent of women are extremely sensitive to ovulation induction medications and experience sometimes serious side effects as a result. OHSS tends to occur more often in patients with many follicles. OHSS can occur before or after egg retrieval and is associated with severe abdominal bloating, nausea, and vomiting.

Oocyte: The medical term for an egg.

PCOS (Polycystic Ovarian Syndrome): One of the most common endocrine disorders in women. Often associated with a high number of antral follicles by ultrasound, irregular menstrual cycles, and symptoms of elevated androgens such as acne or increased hair growth. Not all factors are necessary for diagnosis. PCOS can be associated with other medical conditions like obesity and diabetes.

PGT or PGT-A (Preimplantation Genetic Testing for Aneuploidy): Preimplantation genetic testing (PGT) is done by sampling/biopsying four to ten cells from the trophectoderm (outer part of the embryo that becomes the placenta) of a day five to six embryo in order to perform genetic testing on the embryo. The most common type of genetic testing is PGT-A (preimplantation genetic testing for aneuploidy). This testing has also been called chromosomal screening (CS) or preimplantation genetic screening (PGS). This test is to see if the embryo has the correct number of chromosomes necessary to produce a healthy baby, which can help in selecting which embryo to transfer to the uterus. The goal is to look for the embryo that will have the highest chance of resulting in a healthy pregnancy and live birth. It is an embryo selection tool that can reduce the risk of miscarriage.

PRL (Prolactin): A hormone in the body that is often called the "breastfeeding hormone." If prolactin levels are high outside of the setting of pregnancy or breastfeeding, there may be negative implications for ovulation or implantation. This value is sometimes checked during a fertility evaluation.

P4 (Progesterone): P4 is an important hormone involved in the menstrual cycle and pregnancy. Progesterone blood levels spike after ovulation occurs. If implantation or pregnancy results, the corpus luteum will continue to produce progesterone to maintain the endometrial lining and support early pregnancy. If pregnancy does not occur, progesterone levels will drop, and the lining will shed with the start of a new menstrual cycle. Progesterone is also a medication sometimes given as part of an IVF cycle or embryo transfer cycle protocol.

REI (Reproductive Endocrinology and Infertility): A reproductive endocrinologist is a fertility doctor who is board certified in reproductive endocrinology and infertility. This means they are fellowship trained and have passed the strictest examinations in the field.

TSH (Thyroid-Stimulating Hormone): A hormone produced by the pituitary gland that stimulates the thyroid to produce thyroid hormones. TSH is a marker of thyroid function and is often part of a routine fertility workup.

TTC (Trying to Conceive): A common abbreviation used in the fertility community when trying for pregnancy.

TVA (Transvaginal Aspiration): Eggs are collected (retrieved) by ultrasound-guided needle aspiration through the vagina. A needle is used to gently suck the fluid out of each follicle. With the fluid comes the eggs. The medical term for an egg retrieval is transvaginal oocyte aspiration because the aspiration of the eggs happens via a needle through the vaginal wall.

About the Authors

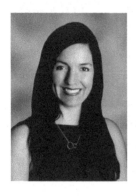

Julie Lamb, MD, FACOG, is a board certified reproductive endocrinologist and infertility specialist at Pacific NW Fertility in Seattle.

Dr. Lamb graduated at the top of her medical school class at Northwestern University Feinberg School of Medicine in Chicago. She was awarded a Fulbright Scholarship to study international women's health in Zimbabwe. Dr. Lamb completed her residency in obstetrics and gynecology at the University of Washington in Seattle and did her fellowship in reproductive endocrinology and infertility at University of California, San Francisco. As clinical faculty at the University of Washington, she directs the REI training of Ob/Gyn resident physicians and is the director of the Center for Fertility Preservation at Pacific NW Fertility.

Dr. Lamb is committed to combining state of the art technology and exceptional patient care to help patients meet their family building goals. She has presented and published over 50 peer-reviewed research projects at national meetings and is an active board member of both the American Society for Reproductive Medicine patient education committee and embryo transfer committee and Pacific Coast Reproductive Society. She is also past president of Seattle Gynecologic Society.

Dr. Lamb is dedicated to changing the conversation surrounding fertility care and strives to empower women to learn about their fertility and their options. She also enjoys cycling, skiing, camping, and spending time with friends and family.

Emily Gray, RN, BSN, was born
and raised in the greater Seattle area
and attended nursing school at
Gonzaga University in Spokane,
Washington. Emily is now living in
Seattle with her husband, Phil, and
works at Pacific NW Fertility as an
IVF coordinator and director of IVF
nursing. From a very early age, Emily
felt drawn to the world of
reproductive medicine, including the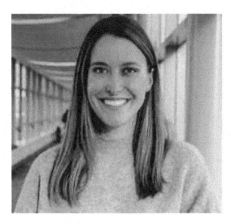
science behind this fascinating field, the psychology involved, and the
impact reproduction has on individuals and couples from all walks of
life. Emily has a passion for patient and nursing education and finds
true joy from working alongside patients during one of the most
difficult and personal times in their lives.

Acknowledgements

We would like to thank Dr. Lamb's lovely friend, Michelle "Mitch" Peterson (mitchdorsey@yahoo.com), for the female reproductive art on the cover and title page. She is a true talent, and we know she will continue to inspire and empower women through her work.

A thank you also to Dr. Lamb's sister, Renee Hwang, for her beautiful work on the cover and to our amazing editor, Lucy Elenbaas, who pulled everything together and helped make this book possible every step of the way.

We would like to also thank our incredible team at Pacific NW Fertility (PNWF), who day after day take the best possible care of each patient, each egg, and each embryo. We are so grateful to work with each of you!

And of course, many thanks to our husbands, Andrew and Phil, for the unrelenting love and support for all we do.

Made in USA - Kendallville, IN
75049_9781792340840
05.04.2022 1314